Understanding
Your
Medical
Laboratory Tests
and
Surgical
Biopsy Reports

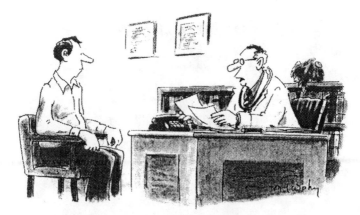

"I'll want to run a few tests on you, just to cover my ass."

Understanding Your Medical Laboratory Tests and Surgical Biopsy Reports

A Patient's Guide

Imprimatur:
Martin Meadow Press

Robert W. Christie, M.D., FCAP, FASCP
Auctor ignotus

Xlibris.com   Philadelphia

Copyright © 2005 by Robert W. Christie M.D.

Library of Congress Number: 2005901955
ISBN :   Hardcover   1-4134-4731-7
                Softcover   1-4134-4730-9

This book was printed in the United States of America.

Design: Robert W. Christie M.D.,
        Junico A. and Jessfer C.—Xlibris Designers

To order additional copies of this book, contact:
Xlibris Corporation
1-888-795-4274
www.Xlibris.com
Orders@Xlibris.com

20002

Other books by the author

Actions and Decisions:
Concise Consultations for the Clinical Pathologist*

Fate's Finger**

Indigenous Design:
Fascinating Signs Along Highways and Byways**

A Greenland Journal

Wooden Props, Canvas Wings

*Published by and available from ASCP Press
**Published by and available from www.Xlibris.com

CONTENTS

Acknowledgements 15
Preface 17

I

Understanding Your Medical Laboratory Tests and Test Reports

Foreword.. 21

Chapter 1: It's YOUR Blood!:
The Empowerment of the Patient 23

Chapter 2: Choosing Tests to
Meet Your Health Worries 29

Chapter 3: Test Results: Normal, Decision,
and Action Levels 36

Chapter 4: The Role of the
Laboratory Test in Diagnosis 44

Chapter 5: What You Should Expect in a
Laboratory Test Report 56

Chapter 6: Numbers and Normal Ranges 67

Chapter 7: Preparation for Laboratory Tests 70

Chapter 8: Direct Access Testing 72

Chapter 9: Interpretation Formats, Tests for
Symptoms and Worries, and
Normal Values for Tests 78

II

Understanding Your Surgical Biopsy Report

Foreword 95

Chapter 10: Your Surgical Pathology Biopsy Report 97

III

Interpretations of Medical Laboratory Test Results

Foreword 109

Chapter 11: Acute Disease Tests 111

Chapter 12: Annual Check-up Tests 148

Chapter 13: Blood Disease Tests 173

Chapter 14: Cancer Screening Tests 197

Chapter 15: Chronic Disease Tests 212

Chapter 16: Heart Disease Tests 261

Chapter 17: Infant, Child and
Adolescent Screening Tests 276

Chapter 18: Legal-issue Tests 288

Chapter 19: Libido Test 295

Chapter 20: Menopause Tests 299

Chapter 21: Pregnancy and Infertility Tests 303

Chapter 22: Prostate Disease Tests 321

Chapter 23: Sexually Transmitted Disease (STD)
Tests 330

Chapter 24: Therapeutic Drug Monitoring Tests 341

Afterword 357

Index 361

Dedication

To those patients who are so intimidated by
"white coat" authoritarianism that they don't dare
ask their doctor questions.

"The era of physicians' monopoly of medical facts and practices is over, and well it should be. Medical imperialism is obsolete."

Jerome P. Kassirer, M.D.
Former Editor, *The New England Journal of Medicine*

Editorial: Practicing Medicine Without a License—
The New Intrusion by Congress.
N Eng J Med 1997; 336:1747

Advance Praise

"Congratulations for comprehending the difficulty the non-medical person has in understanding reports from a medical laboratory or a surgeon's office—and doing something about it!"
David S. Dana, Automotive Industry executive

"A great resource for the lay population . . . . and everyone who works at our Clinic should have a copy of this humorous, incisive look into the mysterious world of lab tests!"
Penny Durgin, A.D.N.P., Nurse Practitioner

"Great idea for a book! I'm sure it will be a great help to patients trying to interpret their lab test results, and it will surely be an aid to medical caretakers in discussing test reports with their patients—and it will be on my bookshelf!"
Elwin Falkenham, M.D., Family Practitioner

". . . . the explanations of the lab tests make for fast, easy reading. I hope many doctors and nurse practitioners will read it and learn a few things they really need to know in dealing with apprehensive patients—like me."
Annette McMahon, High School teacher

"The reach of the subject of laboratory testing is really comprehensive. A reader can go to whatever depth he or she chooses; many will find satisfaction in the informal style and avoidance of medical language that is incomprehensible to patients."

John L. Meyer II, M.D., FASCP,
Community hospital Pathologist

"I have read Dr. Christie's book with great interest and pleasure. He is absolutely right about the communications gap between patient and doctor, and so this book will appeal to a large audience, particularly the worried well, who comprise a large part of the population and of every doctor's practice."

James Russell, M.D., Internist

"I love it! This book is an important resource for the public. The definitions are very clear. This will be well received by all those people who love to know about their health problems (I'm one of them). Members of the legal profesion will find useful information here too."

Anne F. Ward, Attorney

"Using this book, patients will be able to understand the significance of their laboratory tests results. So often explanations from doctors in their offices are too hurried, too technical, and too upsetting for patients to comprehend what their tests really mean."

April Whithed, MT(ASCP), Laboratory Manager

ACKNOWLEDGEMENTS

I am indebted to and most grateful for the advice, suggestions, criticisms, and encouragement from Glenn Adams, D.O., Emilie Burack, Mary Burack, Richard Burack, M.D., Elaine and David Dana, Nancy Dixon, Penny Durgin, A.D.N.P., Elwin Falkenham, M.D., the late Freeman Keith, Annette McMahon, John L. Meyer II, M.D., James Russell, M.D., Roderick Stinehour, Anne F. Ward, and April Whithed, MT (ASCP).

All, each in their own realm of expertise, were most helpful in bringing encouragement, suggestions, and constructive criticism to the author in the writing and design of this venture into the world of consumer information.

The author also wishes to congratulate Mike Twohy for his marvelous insight into the workings of the medical mind, exhibited on the cover and frontispiece of this book. Touché, Mike!

PREFACE

Are you worried about cancer, heart attacks, or have other health concerns? Are you confused or bewildered by the terms used in the pathologist's report to your surgeon about a recent biopsy or operation? If you are, you are not alone. Laboratory test results are often thought by patients to be mysterious, secret or coded information for doctors' and nurses' eyes only. After all, it's your blood (or urine, or body cells, or whatever else is being tested) and you are entitled to know what's been found!

This should not be the case in the world of communication in which we live. Here, in patient understandable language, you will find out which laboratory tests you should have to resolve your worrisome symptoms or health concerns, what the test report numbers mean, whether your test results are abnormal, and if so, what actions you should take. You will also find a chapter on the meaning of the terms and tests referred to in surgical pathology reports relating to commonly biopsied tissues such as bone marrow, breast, cervix, colon, lymph nodes, prostate and skin.

Were you aware that in many laboratories in this and other countries you can order your own tests and get the test results yourself without going through a doctor's office twice to get the information? You can find out about that in this book too.

The book is in three parts: Part I, *Understanding Laboratory Tests and Test Reports,* Part II, *Understanding Your Surgical Biopsy*

Report, and Part III, *Interpretations of Laboratory Test Results.* You will find here the normal values for commonly ordered tests, discover which tests your primary care doctor or nurse practitioner should be ordering when you have your periodic health check-up, and what you—and your doctor—should expect to find in a meaningful and understandable laboratory report.

But here is a warning. Laboratory science is always evolving. Newer, better, faster laboratory tests continually emerge. New discoveries, new insights, and revised understanding of former knowledge will always displace what formerly has been accepted as the truth, for often this truth is only "the current wisdom" that later will be shown to be incorrect as scientific inquiry progresses. Furthermore, not all professionals agree on every subject, which is very important and fortunate for the continuous advancement of scientific medicine. Without disagreement and debate, scientific inquiry and human progress wither and die. A basic tenet of scientific inquiry is to continually absorb, suspect, doubt, challenge, and debate what is printed in scientific journals and books—including this one.

Perhaps the most important message in this guide is to encourage individuals to take more personal responsibility for their health and wellness by learning and understanding more about what's going on inside their bodies through laboratory testing, before irreversible changes occur. With this knowledge, patients (consumers!) can become active and informed partners with their healthcare providers rather than passive recipients of healthcare services—and live longer, healthier lives.

I

*Understanding Your
Medical Laboratory
Tests and Test Reports*

FOREWORD

This section provides general background information about medical laboratory testing, its importance in finding out what is going on inside your body—information usually not disclosed by a physical examination of the outside of your body.

CHAPTER 1

It's *YOUR* Blood!:

The Empowerment of the Patient

No one lives forever, but no one wants to die unnecessarily soon either. All of us who are aware of the need to develop good health habits are also aware that it is almost always far better to detect disease early rather than late. Many fear cancer, HIV infection and AIDS, sexually transmitted diseases, diabetes, heart attacks, urinary tract infections, infertility, strep throats, and a myriad of other illness. So to varying extents we each, depending on our personal or family health history, our personality and our neuroses, are always checking our own health status. Laboratory tests play a large role in uncovering clues to unsuspected disease.

We get up in the morning and check our health status by looking in the mirror. This is a "direct-access test" to see how we look, a quick and casual assessment of our health. We go through our daily fifteen-second check-up. This speedy evaluation tells us bluntly or subtly whether we think we are in good shape or not. It's analogous to the quick "systems review" the physician does.

The conversation with oneself before the mirror might go like this:

> "Maybe my eyes are a little blood-shot. Conjunctivitis? Probably not; just not enough sleep or too much to drink last night. Grey hair and wrinkles are about the same as yesterday; not aging too fast. Runny nose, must have picked up a virus; maybe it will have dried up by breakfast. Skin looks scaly on the hands; maybe too much sun exposure, should use sunscreen more often. Belly sticks out too far. Looks better when I pull it in. Maybe I need to go on a diet again; everyone knows it's not good for your heart to be overweight. Hmm, tongue looks coated; better use some mouthwash, get rid of the germs. Corn on my left foot looks a little bigger. Maybe that needs some trimming. Well, I'm probably in pretty good shape for my age. Time for my shower. Maybe I'll make an appointment at the Clinic next week and get a couple of lab tests done, just to make sure everything's okay".

Many of us are among the "worried well". In the medical profession that's the label for a person who isn't sick by medical standards, but who fears an imagined illness of any sort, and worries about it enough to see a physician or other health-care provider. The "worried well" is an excellent expression—it describes those of us who are perhaps unduly concerned about our health, maybe because of continual bombardment from the media on health issues. There have been suggestions that as much as 40% of an internist's or family practitioner's practice is devoted to the worried well. Many of these worried well are more and more frequently assigned to physician's assistants or nurse practitioners for attention in order to free the physician to spend more time with those who are truly and observably ill and need immediate medical care.

And because doctors like to please their patients, they often order medical tests to reassure the patient that his or her suspected illness doesn't exist. This rarely works for long for the worried well patient, but it gives both doctor and patient the feeling that something is being done. Of course the problem is that the worried well are also mortal; sometimes their worries *are* well founded. Check-up laboratory tests sometimes *do* uncover something important, so ordering tests also protects the doctor from liability if, as occasionally occurs, the worried well patient really does have something seriously wrong that has been overlooked or dismissed because the patient perhaps has cried wolf too often. This needs no amplification here. The frontispiece in this book from the *The New Yorker* magazine says it all.

In my opinion, Dr. Jerome Kassirer, a former editor of *The New England Journal of Medicine* is "right on". In an editorial in that prestigious journal he stated: "The era of physicians' monopoly of medical facts and practices is over, and well it should be. Medical imperialism is obsolete. Physicians should no more have exclusive dominion over medical information and decisions than attorneys should have control over the facts and the practice of the law."

The author recently received a letter from an old American friend living in Israel, perhaps a valetudinarian, whose experience with a doctor epitomized the concept of "medical imperialism":

> "Went to the Doctor this week, ready to die. He fixed it in one shot for $3.00. So I asked: "What do I have?
> The Doctor said, "*Garnisht mit garnisht.*"

According to my friend, the term "*garnisht*" derives from the German "*garnichts*", meaning in English "nothing". It sounds as though medical imperialism also prevails in the Middle East—and perhaps worldwide if one may extrapolate from a base of two. Apparently, the message that "medical imperialism is obsolete" hasn't gotten beyond Boston, yet. But at least my friend's doctor didn't feel the need to run a few lab tests, and my friend is still alive and well.

And this leads us to what perhaps is a new era in laboratory testing, the era of DAT. In current laboratory jargon, "DAT" is the acronym and buzzword for "Direct Access Testing", the ability of a patient to order his or her own laboratory tests without going through a doctor to get an order for the tests. Direct access testing is just a variation of what we do by looking at ourselves in the mirror every day; these tests look at what's going on inside our body. But laboratory tests are a lot more difficult to obtain and certainly are more expensive than a soliloquy in front of the mirror. In effect, DAT is an extension of health self-appraisals by an individual before, or at the time, he or she becomes a patient with a real symptom, complaint, or illness.

Experience tells us, of course, that most laboratory test results turn out to be "normal", not abnormal. No one knows what percentage of the population out there actually has blood in the stool, or a high blood sugar, or a fetus with a genetic defect growing within the mother's uterus. But for most of us, it would be nice—I would argue essential—to know, one way or the other, if things are really okay inside our bodies.

Right now, over-the-counter (OTC) testing is prevalent in most technologically-oriented societies to augment the in-front-of-the-mirror daily health appraisal. Anyone can buy a pregnancy test kit, urine test strips, test strips for checking blood sugar levels, and many other similar items. Measuring instruments the likes of digital thermometers, digital reading bathroom scales, automatic-inflating and digital-recording blood pressure devices with pulsimeters are all available to those who have a need to know what their bodies are doing compared to some standard they or their doctor may have set for themselves. They must only be willing to pay the price to have them from a pharmacy or elsewhere.

However, if you want to know what your blood sugar has been for the last few weeks ("there's a family history of diabetes on Mom's side"), or whether that ache in your big toe means gout (you've heard that blood uric acid is high if you have gout), or if you want a cholesterol test (to forewarn you of any likelihood that you might have a heart attack), you discover that you can only have the blood tests you would like to have performed by getting a doctor's order—and that means you have to go to the doctor or nurse practitioner, whose office hours often happen to coincide with the hours you must be at work.

And then there are other roadblocks. You find that your doctor takes patients only by appointment, and he or she is booked up for three weeks. And it may cost $35.00—often far more—just to get to see the doctor—if your employer is agreeable to your being away from your job for several hours. And then, unless of course there just happens to be a laboratory in the doctor's office, your doctor is apt to say, "Why do you think you need that?" perhaps in an intimidating tone of voice. You feel foolish, frustrated and put down, while your doctor feels his authority is being challenged by some nincompoop who has just read an article in *Cosmopolitan* or a health letter about the need for everyone to have a test for serum rhubarb to uncover a possible latent subacute omphalitis (translation: could be an unsuspected, waiting-to-happen smoldering infection of the belly button).

If the doctor is cooperative, you will probably get your test, and perhaps one or several more that you never thought or heard of. Of course, the test results will go only to the doctor, and not to you, who really wants the information, and who pays for the test. Later, when you get the note from your health insurance carrier you discover to your dismay that no one told you that the tests are not covered under your policy ("*see denial code 17*"). Now you have a big laboratory bill on your hands as well as another doctor's appointment. That will not be free either.

But there is more to it than the economics: there is the issue of personal responsibility, to care for ourselves instead of passing accountability on to a health care provider. That's what this book is about—how to understand what laboratory test results mean in relation to your concern for your own well being; how to get clinical laboratory tests results from a reliable laboratory directly, without the hassle, the frustration, the lost time from work—and two doctor's bills; and to find out what the test results mean in terms of keeping well or prompting one to seek medical care. In short, it is an empowerment of the individual so he or she will take more responsibility for his or her health and well-being. Remember Dr. Kassirer's remark: "Medical imperialism is obsolete"—whether in Boston or Tel Aviv.

And also remember: you are *entitled* to ask for laboratory tests, to be given access to the test results, to be told what the test results mean in terms of your health, and to find out what action, if any, must be taken for follow-up. You, or your employer has *paid* for the tests.

And after all—it's *YOUR* body; it's *YOUR* blood!

CHAPTER 2

Choosing Tests to

Meet Your Health Worries

A s the old Dutchman said, "He who has a choice has trouble!" There are thousands of medical laboratory tests that can be performed, but only a small percentage of these are available at most clinical laboratories. Hospital laboratories have a menu of tests available roughly in proportion to the size of the hospital. However, through the use of reference laboratories, even smaller clinical laboratories have access to a very large number of tests. But which tests are important to the person who is concerned about a health matter? That depends entirely on what one is concerned or worried about.

There is no point in ordering laboratory tests that will not produce information that can be used intelligently to solve a problem or to alleviate a concern or worry. Common worries or concerns and some appropriate tests to help resolve them are shown in Table 1. It is important to be aware, however, that the tests listed in the Table are not the *only* tests that might be selected by a physician, but are tests generally accepted as applicable to a possible cause for your worry. For example, depression is only very occasionally caused by hypothyroidism, and obtaining a normal thyroid test result has only eliminated one possible organic cause for the depression; also, only rarely is hypertension caused by an adrenal gland tumor that might be detected by measuring metanephrines.

Table 1

Laboratory Tests Addressing
Common Patient Health Concerns

SYMPTOMS or WORRIES	TEST	COST ($US)*
AIDS or HIV	HIV test	64.00
ALCOHOL	Blood alcohol	68.00
	(to establish sobriety)	
ANEMIA	Complete blood count	25.00
	Hemoglobin/hematocrit	21.00
	Serum iron	29.00
	Cyanocobalamin (Vitamin B12)	68.00
	Anemia profile, basic	136.00
ARTHRITIS	Rheumatoid arthritis (RA) test	34.00
	Lupus erythematosus (LE) test	33.00
	Arthritis profile	156.00
	C-Reactive protein	42.00
CERVICAL CANCER	Pap smear **	27.00
COLON CANCER	Stool for occult (hidden) blood	25.00
CYSTIC FIBROSIS (CF)	Chloride Sweat Test	(NA)
	Cystic Fibrosis DNA Content	
	(if there is a family history of CF)	(NA)
DEPRESSION	Thyroid Stimulating Hormone (TSH)	85.00
DIABETES	Fasting plasma glucose (FBS)	10.00
DIARRHEA	Stool for Ova and Parasites	100.00
	Stool culture	59.00

DRUG MONITORING	Lithium	39.00
	Theophylline	67.00
	Phenytoin (Dilantin)	69.00
	Salicylate (Aspirin)	55.00
	Digoxin	47.00
	Prothrombin Time (PT)	26.00
EASY BRUISING	Platelet Count (PC)	21.00
	Prothrombin time (PT)	26.00
	Activ. partial thromboplastin time (APTT)	47.00
ENDOMETRIAL CANCER	Pap smear **	27.00
GIARDIASIS	Stool for Ova and Parasites	100.00
GOUT	Uric acid	27.55
HEART ATTACK RISK (cardiac risk) (HDLC)	Total cholesterol (TC)	27.00
	High density lipoprot.	36.50
	Low density lipoprot. (LDLC)	(NA)
	Cardiac Risk profile group	66.00
	TC:HDLC	(NA)
	Triglycerides	27.00
	Apolipoprotein	81.00
	Homocysteine	140.00
HEART RACING (tachycardia)	Thyroxine (T-4)	32.00
HEMOCHROMATOSIS	Serum iron (too much liver iron)	29.00
HYPERTENSION	Metanephrines, total	87.00
HYPOGLYCEMIA	5 hr. glucose tolerance (GTT-5)	54.00
	(low blood sugar) Blood insulin	(NA)
INFECTIOUS MONO- NUCLEOSIS ("Mono")	Monospot/heterophil antibody	31.00
KIDNEY CANCER	Urinalysis with micro exam	22.00
KIDNEY DISEASE	Renal profile (BUN, Creatinine)	53.00

LEAD POISONING	Blood lead	52.00
LEUKEMIA	Complete Blood Count	25.00
LIVER DISEASE	Hepatitis panel	125.00
LIVER DISEASE (alcoholic)	CBC with RBC Indices Serum Folate	25.00 63.00
LOW BLOOD SUGAR	5 hr. glucose tolerance (GTT-5) (hypoglycemia) Blood insulin	54.00 (NA)
MALE FERTILITY	Semen analysis	81.00
"MONO" (INFECTIOUS MONONUCLEOSIS)	Monospot/heterophil antibody	31.00
OSTEOPOROSIS	Osteocalcin	116.00
OVARIAN CANCER	Carcinoembryonic antigen (CEA)	87.00
PENILE DISCHARGE	HIV Genital Culture RPR for Syphilis Serology	68.00 52.00 41.00
PEPTIC ULCER (stomach ulcer)	*H. pylori* Serology Stool for Occult Blood	85.00 25.00
PREGNANCY	Chorionic gonadotrophin (PHCG) Folic acid (folate) Alpha1 fetoprotein (AFP) , Serum and Amniotic fluid***	43.00 63.00 (NA)
PROSTATE CANCER	Prostate specific antigen (PSA)	88.00
SEXUALLY TRANSMITTED DISEASE (exposure, or vaginal or penile discharge)	HIV test Genital Culture for *Neisseria gonorrheae, Chlamydia trachomatis, Candida albicans* RPR Syphilis Serology Urogenital viral culture	64.00 52.00 41.00 183.00
SORE THROAT	*S. pneumoniae* ("Strep Screen") Heterophil/Monospot Throat culture	31.00 31.00 49.00

STOMACH ULCER	*H. pylori* Serology	85.00
(peptic ulcer)	Stool for Occult Blood	25.00
THYROID PROBLEM	Thyroid stimulating hormone (TSH)	85.00
	Thyroxine (T-4)	33.00
TIRED or COLD ALL	Thyroid stimulating hormone	85.00
THE TIME (TSH)	Blood lead	52.00
	Complete Blood Count	25.00
URINARY BURNING	Urine culture	43.00
or FREQUENCY	Blood culture	64.00
	Urinalysis	22.00
VAGINAL DISCHARGE	Genital Culture	52.00
WEIGHT LOSS	Thyroxine (T-4)	33.00

*   Source: commercial reference laboratory; *exempletive only: costs of tests varies widely amongst laboratories and change over time.*

**   not all laboratories have facilities for vaginal Pap smear preparation.

***   requires special collection techniques by physician; charges vary widely.

(NA): not applicable for various reasons.

Important:

The tests arbitrarily listed above may not be specific for your worry! Your physician may select these or other tests based on your medical history or symptoms and signs of illness. New tests are continually being developed and may not be included in the above table.

This list of almost eighty tests presents a manageable menu of choices for the consumer from the thousands of tests available. It does not mean to imply that there aren't other worries or concerns, or that those in Table 1 are the *only* tests that might be appropriate to alleviate or confirm the worry, but the list does include tests that are readily available from most accredited clinical laboratories.

But what about tests that should be done routinely and periodically, as when you have your annual physical check-up with your doctor? Yes, there are some tests called *screening tests* (Table 2), that is, tests that may pick up evidence of a disease or syndrome that is developing but has not yet produced any physical signs or symptoms. These are the tests most internists, family practitioners, pediatricians, or nurse practitioners usually order to round out their appraisal of your health, or the health of your child.

Table 2

Important Health Appraisal Screening Tests

TEST	WHO	WHY	HOW OFTEN
Urinalysis	All	Screens for urinary tract infections or bleeding; diabetes	Yearly
Blood sugar	All	Screens for diabetes	Yearly
Cholesterol	All	Screens for likelihood of coronary artery disease	Once before age 20 years; every 3 years thereafter
Complete blood count (CBC)	All	Screens for anemia, leukemia, infections, bleeding disorders	Yearly
Stool for blood	All	Screens for colon cancer, GI bleeding	Yearly

Pap Smear	All female adults	Screens for uterine and vaginal cancer, and infections	Yearly
Blood lead	All children	Screens for lead exposure or lead poisoning	Yearly to at least age 5 years
Prostate	All men 50 years and older	Prostate cancer specific antigen (PSA)*	Yearly
TSH	All	Hypothyroidism	Yearly after age 70

Discuss with your doctor.

The number of screening tests for health appraisal in Table 2 is short, a "bare bones" list, because it includes screening tests that have proven to be both cost-effective and useful over the years for picking up unsuspected disease early, before a medical crisis has occurred or before it is too late for disease control or a cure.

Some doctors may order more tests than those listed in Table 2 at the time of an "annual physical", but in the author's opinion, none should order fewer. One must keep in mind, of course, that other laboratory tests (as well as other types of tests, e.g., a mammogram) may be ordered to confirm or rule out anything your health examiner uncovers during his or her routine check-up examination.

If your healthcare provider has overlooked or neglected to order any of the screening tests in Table 2, you have a right to—and should ask for—an explanation. If you are not satisfied with the response, you have three courses of action. You can persuade your doctor to order those tests that you know you should have, you can find another doctor who does believe in the worth of screening tests such as those listed above, or you can look for a laboratory that offers direct access testing (*see Chapter 9*).

CHAPTER 3

Test Results: Normal, Decision, and

Action Levels

U nless you understand what the terms "normal", or "within normal limits" (WNL) mean for any laboratory test, it is easy to become concerned, confused, alarmed, or indeed panicked. Laboratory test results are always shown on a report related to certain standards. These standards are the average tests results taken from a large group of people who were known to be healthy, free of the diseases that the test is designed to detect. Such standards are referred to as "normal ranges", or in laboratory parlance, "reference ranges". There are reference ranges for almost all laboratory tests, and these are always shown with your test result numbers.

It is important to know that reference ranges are not chiseled into granite. As new epidemiological knowledge becomes available concerning certain diseases, tighter or looser limits for the ranges may be established. This has happened occasionally with regard to blood sugar test limits, where different ranges have been established for subsets of the population, for instance the limits for a pregnant woman's or a newborn infant's blood sugar.

Physicians usually repond to laboratory test data at three levels: normal, decision, and action. Here we will look at each of these levels.

1. *Normal Test Results: a reason to rejoice*

Let's take an example. You or your doctor have asked the laboratory to test your blood for sugar because there is diabetes in your family or because of certain symptoms you have; here is your test result:

Blood Glucose: 100 mg/dL (reference range 60-110 mg/dL).

A blood glucose test measures the amount of a certain type of sugar in a specific amount of blood that has been removed from your bloodstream. The type of sugar is glucose. The amount (weight) of glucose is expressed in *milligrams ("mg")*. The amount of blood (volume) is one (1) *deciliter ("dL")*, which is one tenth of a liter (one liter is about equivalent to one quart). Many laboratories now use *millimols ("mmol")* instead of milligrams for some chemistry tests, but *"mg"* and *"mmol"* mean essentially the same thing.

Is 100 mg/dL normal? To know this, it is necessary to study what the blood glucose is in a large number of healthy people. This has been done, and the information discovered is very well known. In people who are not diabetic and otherwise in good health the blood glucose falls somewhere on or between 60 mg/dL and 115 mg/dL. The 60 is called the "lower limit", and the 115 the "upper limit" of the normal range of the test. Test results on or between the numbers 60 and 115 are considered to be, and are variously termed, "within the reference range", "within normal range", "within normal limits" ("WNL"), or just "normal". All these terms mean the same thing.

In this example, the blood glucose is 100 mg/dL. Since it falls between 60 and 115, it is within the reference (normal) range, and so is considered "normal". This means that you do not have a disease associated with abnormally high blood glucose such as diabetes mellitus, or hypoglycemia (low blood glucose) caused by some other disease or medication.

Of course, there a few other things that have to be considered. The blood test for sugar had to be performed under some fairly standard conditions, because the reference range was established by testing healthy people under identical conditions. These conditions would include being within a certain age bracket, and not having eaten or drunk anything for several hours before the blood was obtained. For the generally accepted reference ranges for frequently ordered tests, see Part III, *Interpretations of Medical Laboratory Test Results* further on in this book.

All numerically expressed laboratory test results have reference ranges, but test results just a little bit above or a little bit below the numbers defining the reference range occasionally happen. Suppose the blood glucose test result is 58 mg/dL, a little below the limits of the reference range, or 118 mg/dL, a little above. These minor deviations, one to three percent beyond the reference range, usually would be of no concern, and ordinarily would not indicate that the test needed to be repeated for confirmation. My own physician refers to these just-out-of-normal-range test results as "wobbles" and usually disregards them as insignificant abnormalities.

A valid reason for receiving a marginal test result such as 58 or 118 might be that the laboratory could have been turning out test results on everyone's blood that are just a little bit low or a little bit high that day. This is unlikely in a well-run laboratory, but bad laboratory days (like "bad hair days") do happen, and if the day your test was run turns out to be one of those days, the laboratory has a responsibility to let you know that in their report to you. A more common reason is that because humans are biologically complex, something may be going on within one's body that alters the test results. An example would be having a fever, or being pregnant at the time the blood sample was obtained.

If you have questions about slightly aberrant test results, call your physician. Interpretation of laboratory test results is an art that may require medical judgment, even when the results seem to be normal. It is often not known or forgotten by healthcare providers of all kinds that the reference range for a test may vary because of your age, weight, sex, medications and drugs you are taking, your nutritional state, your circadian rhythm, recent exercise, and even your posture when the specimen is collected.

2. Decision Test Results: a reason for concern

It is a pleasant fact that most laboratory test results are normal. That is, they fall on or between numbers in the reference range for the test. Steady trends in test results even within the normal range are, however, quite useful in diagnosis if they show a progression over time in the same direction, either higher or lower. Test results on spreadsheet formatted reports are quite useful for demonstrating trends over time, but presently few laboratories employ them.

It is when test results are somewhat outside of the reference range that some decisions must be made. As has been mentioned before, if test results are within the reference range there is nothing to do other than rejoice. It is when they are at a decision (or action) level that something should happen. Decision levels are test results which would perhaps make a physician raise his eyebrows, if not purse his lips upon reading a report.

If your test result is at a decision level, as indicated on a properly designed laboratory report, a physician should be consulted to evaluate your symptoms and/or abnormal signs of disease, if you happen to have either or both of these. Because many laboratory test abnormalities are not accompanied by any demonstrable changes in health however, your physician may want to delve deeper into your medical history, make a review of your body systems and your health habits, and then either do what is called "watchful waiting", or order more tests. Often it will be the latter, to clarify the muddy waters of a differential diagnosis. All too frequently, because of the Damoclesian sword of a possible malpractice lawsuit hanging over the heads of physicians, there will be another reason, made clear in a the cartoon in *The New Yorker* magazine used as a frontispiece for this book. Whatever the physician decides, the ball is now both legally and ethically in the doctor's court, and you will presumably follow his or her advice. Your health may be at peril if you do not do so.

3. Action ("Panic") Test Results: a call for immediate action

Action levels are those that would provoke an "Uh-oh!", from your physician rather than raised eyebrows or pursed lips. When laboratory test results fall far out of the reference range, they are sometimes referred to as "panic values". A panic value implies that there is something that someone should be in a panic, or at least very concerned, about. Just where this term originated is obscure, but it likely was coined by some laboratory technologist who was responsible for doing something about very abnormal test results he or she had just produced.

Action levels are equivalent to panic values. The necessary response to action values is to do something right away, such as initiating treatment, stopping a medication, or perhaps taking out an appendix. Unlike decision-level responses that tend to be more of a "let's wait and see" or—more likely— "let's order more laboratory tests", the action-level response must be more immediate.

So that every laboratory technologist will know whether a test represents a panic value or not, every well-run laboratory has a prominently posted list of panic values for commonly ordered laboratory tests. A laboratorian, upon discovering that a test value is unusually high or low, will refer to this list of panic test results and then will call the patient's physician. The laboratorian then documents that the physician or the physician's surrogate has indeed been notified that the patient has a serious problem of some sort, at least from the laboratory's point of view.

If ever your laboratory test results are at an action level, the situation is immediately urgent. You should call your physician or alternate healthcare provider immediately to discuss the results of your test. The physician will take over from there, possibly (although usually not) instructing you to report to his or her office or the nearest hospital or emergency facility. By no means should you ignore the urgency of the situation, because to do so could be catastrophically dangerous to your well being, perhaps even to your life.

But what if action laboratory test results are given directly to one of the worried well who has gotten his test results after ordering them by direct access testing *(see Chapter 8)*? This problem can easily be resolved in the design of the laboratory test report form, which should have indicated on it the reference ranges for the test as well as an indication of whether the rest results are high, low, or normal. Many laboratory test instruments automatically print out this information beside the test results, usually with an "H" for high and "L" for low test results. A well-designed report form should also have decision level and action level values indicated, so that the recipient of the test result information would be alerted to the need to do something—to get in touch with the family doctor, or other appropriate source of medical information and advice. The telephone number of the patient, and, if the patient wishes, the healthcare provider to be called would usually be asked for when a patient arrives at a laboratory for testing.

An example of an abnormal test result, which would surely generate a call to a patient's doctor if the test were ordered by the doctor from a hospital laboratory, would be a glucose (blood sugar) test value of 27 mg/dL. The reference range for this test in many laboratories (ranges vary slightly from laboratory to laboratory) would be 60-115 mg/dL. While there are a number of causes for a blood sugar this low, the most common cause is overdose of insulin in a diabetic patient. Since the blood test result represents only a single test at one specific time, it is always necessary to know whether the blood sugar is on the way up, or on the way down. At 27 mg/dL it is already bad news; if it is found to be lower at the time of a subsequent test, panic may indeed set in with the clinician, because diabetic insulin shock can be lethal. On the other hand, if, say, the patient's next test result is 43 mg/dL following the intravenous administration of glucose, this is evidence that while all is not yet salubrious, things at least are not getting worse, and probably are improving.

Fortunately, most laboratory test results are not panic values. Perhaps 90% of all laboratory test results are within the reference range. Of the remaining 10%, most are decision-level results. Only about 0.5% or less may represent action-level panic results.

The Problem of False Positives and False Negatives

Occasionally a test result will not mean what the report indicates. This may be a *false positive* or a *false negative*. In a false positive report, it is stated that the results are out of the normal range, but everything else does not confirm that there is anything abnormal or that any disease is present. Rarely, false positives are due to a laboratory mistake; more often they occur because the patient was not properly prepared for the test (e.g., had a drink with high sugar content just before the blood was drawn for a fasting blood sugar test, or had taken a medication that affected one of the body's enzyme systems), or simply because of vagaries of individual physiology (e.g., diurnal rhythm). When a false positive test result is suspected by a patient's doctor, it is usually good practice to repeat the test at a later time under controlled conditions. If the results are still abnormal, the test may be disclosing a real problem that warrants further investigation.

A false negative test is just the opposite. A test may indicate that there is nothing amiss, while indeed something is wrong within the body. An example of this is the test for occult (hidden) blood in the stool, a sign of internal bleeding and disease somewhere within the gastrointestinal (GI) tract (gut). It is well known to physicians that cancer of the colon is discovered only 30% of the time by using the test—the diagnosis is missed because many tests for occult blood turn out to have been falsely negative for a variety of reasons such as not following dietary instructions before the test, or improper sample collection. Again, if suspicion is high and a positive result is anticipated but the appropriate test result is negative and does not confirm other evidence of a problem, it is prudent for the physician to repeat the test or select an alternative test.

If your test is abnormal but in the decision-level range, some response on your part would be prudent, although not necessarily urgent. Conversely, if it is an action-level result one must be quickly decisive; the appropriate decision would be to immediately call or see a physician. Indeed, your physician would strongly urge you to call him or her were you ever to receive a panic value test result. And the sooner the call, the better. This is an example of where the necessity for taking responsibility for one's own health care should be obvious.

CHAPTER 3

CHAPTER 4

The Role of the

Laboratory Test in Diagnosis

H ave you wondered about some of the jargon doctors slip into conversations about your laboratory tests? Here is straight talk. It's about how a medical or surgical diagnosis is reached, and explains how laboratory tests fit into the big picture of diagnosing disease,. This chapter is about the *differential diagnosis*, the distinction between the *sensitivity* and the *specificity* of a laboratory test, *periodic health screening tests* recommended by authoritative organizations (e.g., American Heart Association, U.S. Department of Health and Human Services, *et al*), and the difference between *test panels* and *test groups*.

The Differential Diagnosis

When you have symptoms and they are disquieting enough to bring you to a doctor's office, your doctor has been trained to sort things out in an orderly way so that as quickly as possible she or he can get to the root of the problem and do something about it. Thomas Huxley, a 19th century biologist, said it succinctly: "The great end of life is not knowledge but action". Your doctor wants to find out whether your symptoms add up to something that can be recognized as a disease or a syndrome to which can be applied an acceptable treatment—or *"garnisht"*, as my friend's doctor in Israel put it as recorded in Chapter 1. To do this, your doctor puts together in his or her mind a list of possible diagnoses that your symptoms might represent. This list is something that has been known in medical circles for many years as a "differential diagnosis".

The differential diagnosis may be very long, or it may be very short. Let's look at a relatively short one. Let us say that you are a woman thirty years old. You feel a need to frequently empty your bladder, and when you do, it stings a little. Next, you note that you are going more often, and it burns every time you empty your bladder. You realize something is wrong. The differential diagnoses—the choices amongst possible causes—are several. Either you have a UTI (urinary tract infection), or something else. The "something else" might include urethritis, cystitis, pyelitis, pyelonephritis, or perhaps a urethral caruncle. The list of things it could be is the differential diagnosis.

To come to the correct diagnosis, each item in the list must be sorted out ("ruled out" is the phrase used by doctors.) However, by far the most common cause of the symptoms you have experienced is cystitis, or a bladder infection; a medical aphorism has it that "common diseases occur commonly". You might choose, or your healthcare provider might urge you, to trot down to the local laboratory and obtain a urinalysis to check that out. If the urine is full of white blood cells, you or the laboratory will want to tell your healthcare provider about it right away so that you get the proper treatment. The provider might tell you to go back to the laboratory and ask for a urine culture and sensitivities to antibiotics of any cultured bacteria. The urine culture, which may take about 24 hours or more, will indicate the proper medication to treat your symptoms. If the treatment fails, other items in the differential diagnosis will have to be addressed, but most of the time that will not be necessary. The problem will have been solved at the lowest expense in the shortest period of time without jeopardizing your health—or your pocketbook. Your doctor may ask you to have another urinalysis a week or ten days after the first one to make sure the infection has cleared up. If the urinalysis is again found to be abnormal, you and your doctor will need to work through other possibilities in the differential diagnosis including other laboratory tests, and possibly other diagnostic studies as well.

Another example of how the differential diagnosis is sorted out is when you wake up in the middle of the night with a pain in your abdomen. It hurts all over. You feel lousy, are nauseated, and you think you have a fever. You take a drink of water, and you want to throw up, but that doesn't happen. You go back to bed, and things haven't gotten any better by morning. You are worried enough to call your doctor, who tells you he will meet you in the Emergency Room right away. That you do.

In the ER your doctor asks a few questions, directed to what doctor's call the "chief complaint". That helps to focus on the problem. Your chief complaint is not nausea; it is not fever; it's a pain in your belly that won't go away. Now that the doctor knows this, he or she can direct questions toward elucidating just what could be causing a pain in your belly. Since you are female, the possibility of a problem relating to your reproductive organs, your uterus, tubes, or ovaries has to be considered. So the doctor wants to know when your last usual menstrual period occurred because the pain may be related to an early pregnancy if you are in the child-bearing era of your life.

Now your doctor wants to know about where the pain is located, whether it comes and goes or is steady; whether it is associated with constipation or diarrhea; what your recent eating experiences have been, and whether you took your temperature with a thermometer. Your doctor now has the makings of a differential diagnosis that could include, among other less likely things:

> acute appendicitis
> a gall bladder attack
> an ectopic pregnancy
> a ruptured ovarian cyst
> acute gastroenteritis
> diverticulosis
> a bladder infection
> pelvic inflammatory disease ("P.I.D.")
> mesenteric lymphadenopathy (inflamed lymph
>   nodes near the intestines)
> porphyria

This is your doctor's initial differential diagnosis.

The next move is to try to sort these out, and find the real cause of your symptoms—the actual diagnosis, so that action can be taken to resolve the problem quickly. This leads to more questions about your eating habits, your sexual activity, and a few apparently off-the-wall questions like whether your urine is sometimes a funny color or has an unusual odor.

Now comes the physical examination, the step that may lead to the correct diagnosis and appropriate therapeutic action. At this point your doctor does a quick general examination, starting at your head and proceeding in a general southerly direction, possibly including your eyes, ears, nose and throat, your neck, your chest, (where a stethoscope is maneuvered fore and aft over the heart and lungs), and then to the site of the chief complaint, your abdomen. By feeling around gently (and sometimes not so gently), it becomes evident that your pain is worse when the examiner's fingers push down in an area in the right lower abdomen known as "McBurney's point". A deeper push at the same place with sudden release of finger pressure makes you say "Ow! That hurt!". To your doctor those words mean "rebound tenderness", a classical sign of peritonitis (inflammation of the inside lining of the abdominal cavity).

The differential diagnosis has quickly narrowed down to six items, from which the right diagnosis again must be separated from the less likely. Your doctor is now probably thinking, this young woman has either:

> acute appendicitis, or
> an ectopic pregnancy, or
> pelvic inflammatory disease, or
> a ruptured ovarian cyst, or
> a urinary tract infection, or
> mesenteric lymphadenopathy.

From the more extended medical history your doctor took before you had to take off all your clothes to be examined, it is clear that you have not missed a menstrual period, that you have not had diarrhea, that your last bowel movement was neither bloody nor black, that you have not recently had any meals in exotic ethnic restaurants, that you do not have a burning sensation when you urinate, and that you have not admitted to sleeping around (and your doctor knows you well enough to know that this is unlikely).

Based on the chief complaint, the information gained about the nature of the symptoms, when and how these began, and how long they have lasted, your doctor is about 95% certain that you have acute appendicitis. But to be even more sure, a pelvic and a rectal examination (to check the uterus, ovaries, and fallopian tubes) needs to be done to pinpoint internally the area of maximum tenderness, pain, or swelling. The pelvic and rectal exams show normal internal organs, and confirm that there is tenderness in the lower right side of the abdomen as noted from probing your pelvis with a finger or two from inside the rectum and the vagina.

This is where the clinical laboratory comes onto the scene. At least three laboratory tests are now in order: a complete blood count (CBC), a urinalysis (UA), and a pregnancy test. When the laboratory reports back the tests results, the urinalysis is found to be entirely normal, the pregnancy test is negative, but your white blood count is above normal, and has a "shift to the left", jargon that means that there are more than the usual number of the kind of white blood cells that can occur when there is an acute bacterial infection.

Now your doctor is 99% certain that you have acute appendicitis. Everything fits: you have the usual symptoms, the pain is in the usual place, your white blood cells show that you have an inflammatory process going on inside you. And a urinary tract infection, an ectopic pregnancy, a ruptured ovarian cyst, colitis, and gastroenteritis have been ruled out, that is, essentially excluded from the differential diagnosis.

Now your doctor does the only proper thing. A surgeon is called to examine you to see if he or she confirms your doctor's impression. You will probably be asked to consent to whatever the surgeon then feels is the proper course of action: to do nothing, or more likely, to take out your appendix even though it may be normal because it is a guaranteed prevention of appendicitis in the future. If there is agreement between the surgeon, your doctor, and you—you have the ultimate responsibility and authority—off to the operating room you go, as soon as possible—but the surgeon will likely tell you that there is a possibility that when the surgical team "gets in there" (meaning when the inside of your belly is being viewed through an incision or a laparoscope), a normal appendix may be found, with perhaps a lot of swollen lymph nodes scattered about (that "mesenteric lymphadenitis" in the differential diagnosis).

The foregoing sequence of events has been pretty straight-forward. On the other hand, a far more difficult differential diagnosis may arise when a patient has many vague complaints that are distributed randomly in time and physical location, and perhaps characterized by complaints such as "just not feeling well", "tired all the time", or having generalized or specifically located weakness of the extremities. Such a differential diagnosis may be complicated by negative or equivocal physical examination findings and laboratory tests that are all normal or are only marginally abnormal. The differential diagnosis may include twenty or thirty diseases or syndromes, depending on what organs or systems seem to be involved. Multiple sclerosis (MS) is such an enigmatic disease, and the diagnosis is sometimes only tediously resolved over time by ruling out all the other diseases or syndromes in the list of differential diagnoses.

Patient symptoms are not the only trigger for a differential diagnosis. Radiologists make up lists of differential diagnoses based on their X-ray, CAT scan, and MRI interpretations, and clinical pathologists make up lists of differential diagnoses based on laboratory test results. Of course not all laboratory tests will generate a differential diagnosis; some tests are specific for a certain organ (e.g., prostate), body fluid component (e.g., antihemophiliac globulin), an antibody (e.g., heterophil, found in infectious mononucleosis), or a toxic substance (e.g., lead).

Contrarily, many laboratory tests do generate a differential diagnosis in the mind of the reviewing physician. An example would be a hemoglobin test result of 9.0 gm/ dL of blood. There are many diseases that might cause a lower than usual hemoglobin in a person. Such a differential diagnosis list might include, to name only a few possibilities:

> recent hemorrhage
> cancer of the colon
> sickle cell disease
> iron deficiency
> pernicious anemia.

The laboratory report, therefore, could include at least a partial differential diagnosis that includes those diagnoses of highest probability based on the information available to the physician responsible for preparing the laboratory test report. What such a report would look like will be found in Chapter 5.

Test Sensitivity and Specificity

Two important terms are helpful in understanding laboratory test results. One of these is *specificity,* and the other is *sensitivity* (not the same as the "sensitivities" associated with cultures for bacteria mentioned before relating to the urine culture). Some tests are *specific* because a positive test result indicates with a high probability that the person has the disease. These tests are like a rifle shot hitting in the center of the target. An example would be the test for HIV (human immunodeficiency virus). If the test is "positive", it is highly probable that the individual is infected; if it is "negative", it is highly unlikely that the individual is infected unless the exposure has been very recent.

Conversely, if a person has an elevated white blood cell count, this is not specific for any particular disease. It means rather that the body has responded to some infection or other cause of inflammation by producing a large number of leukocytes (the white blood cells) in the body. The test can be compared to a shotgun blast—it hits a lot of things. An example would be someone with appendicitis. The appendix is inflamed, but it is not possible to diagnose appendicitis from an elevated white blood cell count without other signs and symptoms of the disease. An elevated WBC would only suggest that there was inflammation somewhere, maybe in the appendix, very possibly somewhere else.

The *sensitivity* of a test is different. Some tests, like the WBC are quite *sensitive;* that is, if inflammation is present, the WBC will usually be elevated, but not always, for it is well known to physicians that elderly patients may have an acute inflammatory process such as appendicitis without the WBC being increased. An analogy can be made between a very sensitive test and a seismograph; a very small disturbance may be detected before an earthquake actually happens.

On the other hand, some tests are not very sensitive at all. A disease may have to be fairly far advanced before the test becomes abnormal or "positive". An example is blood in the urine as an indication of kidney cancer; the tumor might be far advanced before blood appears in the urine. The same can be said about blood in the stool as an indication of colon cancer; the blood may show up only after the cancer has grown large and spread. An analogy would be the automobile that comes to a halt because it is out of oil, even though the dipstick has warned of a low oil level for hundreds of miles before anything happened to indicate that a disaster was about to happen. If the warning had been heeded, the engine wouldn't have seized up, and the disaster would have been averted.

Recommended Periodic Health Screening Tests

Certain laboratory tests have been endorsed by various medical and public health organizations (e.g., American Heart Association, American Cancer Society, U.S. Department of Health and Human Services, Canadian Task Force) as prudent or useful for detecting disease early. Some of these tests are appropriate for one sex, or only for specific age groups. Because there is much controversy on this subject, some of the tests suggested by these health organizations are not accepted as necessary screening tests by all of them. It is a bare bones list. Laboratory tests that have been approved by *most* organizations are listed in Table 3 (a somewhat expanded list, not fully agreed upon by all the previously mentioned organizations has been shown in *Chapter 2, Table 2.*).

Table 3

Some tests that have been agreed upon by various authoritative health organizations for early detection of disease

TEST	WHEN
Blood lead	Yearly from infancy to 5 years
Blood sugar (glucose)	At least once before age 20; every 3-5 years after age 40
Cholesterol	At least once before age 20; every 3-5 years after age 35
Complete blood count	Every 3-5 years
Pap test (*sexually active females*)	Yearly, throughout one's lifetime
Stool for blood	Yearly, after age 40
Urinalysis	At least once before age 20; yearly, after age 40.

Test Panels and Groups

Many laboratories offer menus of tests for specific groups of diseases, often at a reduced price from what the total of the tests in the group would cost if the tests were charged for individually. Examples are "arthritis" groups and "cardiac risk" groups; many others are presently available. A wide variety of disease groups are offered by large hospital and clinic laboratories, as well as by reference laboratories. Many smaller laboratories also offer groups of tests, but usually in smaller numbers. Some of the tests shown in Part III, "Interpretations" are available as test groups (e.g., liver, kidney, cardiac risk, heart attack, complete blood count, arthritis).

The problem is what to do with the results from groups of tests. The more tests in the group, the more opportunity there is for misunderstanding and confusion if, for instance, one test in the group is positive and another test is negative, or all are positive, or all are negative. Well, as the old Dutchman said . . . .

A different type of grouping of tests available from many laboratories is known as "test panels". Whereas test groups are oriented to disease, panels are usually related to a laboratory test instrument's built-in programming. Panels, often called "profiles", are groups of tests produced by a laboratory instrument from a single sample of a body fluid such as blood. The choices of tests are determined by the test instrument's program rather than the patient's specific needs. The panel may consist of a few tests or many—sometimes twenty or more—that are produced automatically. They are designed to cover the landscape. The test results are printed out as a list when the instrument's test cycle is completed.

Test panels are done very efficiently and economically, and twenty tests may be only slightly more costly for the laboratory to produce than a single test. The cost savings are due largely to the frugal use of the reagents needed in testing and great savings in technologist time. These savings are offset by the initial cost of the automated testing instrument, its operational costs, and the overhead costs of the laboratory. But once the instrument has been paid for and is being depreciated in the profit and loss ledger for the laboratory, profit margins can increase considerably. Charges for tests can be changed to reflect this. Thus, it may cost about the same to do a large number of tests—most of them unnecessary but provided anyway—on one sample of body fluid than it costs to do only one or two tests that may be important for a specific diagnosis

Of course that does not mean that the charges to the patient or client will necessarily be lower, but most laboratories will charge for the panel as a unit. Others may charge for the panel at the same rate as the charge for each individual test on the panel. This could result in a bill to the client or patient that can be outrageous. Fortunately, most laboratories offer reduced prices for panels, just as they do for specific test groups.

The good news about panels is that a lot of information is produced for a relatively small cost. The bad news is that most of the test results are of little or no diagnostic help to the client or the doctor and fall into the category of unnecessary tests. Third party payors (and especially the Federal Government), suspecting an opportunity for fraud, do not like to pay for unnecessary tests regardless of why or how they are produced. They may refuse to reimburse a patient or a hospital for such groupings of tests, even though one or more of the test results (whether normal or abnormal) may be relevant to the patient's problem or represent a preventive medical test. So economics and politics creep into this aspect of one's life—just as in every other.

CHAPTER 5

What You Should Expect in a

Laboratory Test Report

One of my relatives recently had a Prostate Specific Antigen (PSA) ordered by his doctor. He was told that the test was being done "to check on the prostate gland", but he had no idea what that meant; he thought it might be a urine test. The test was performed on his blood at a nearby hospital laboratory. Here is what the report that he received in the mail eight days later actually looked like *(all names are fictitious)*:

Illustration 1.

An example of an actual report received by a patient for a Prostate Specific Antigen (PSA) test.

(all proper names are fictitious)

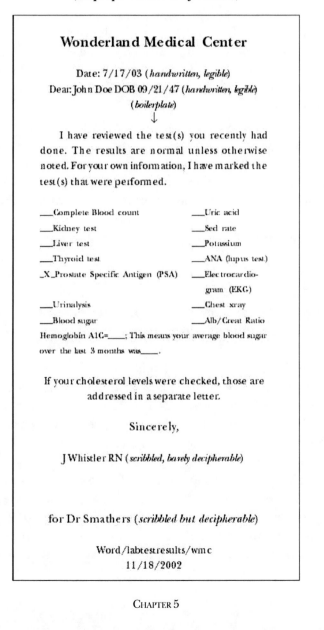

Wonderland Medical Center

Date: 7/17/03 (*handwritten, legible*)
Dear: John Doe DOB 09/21/47 (*handwritten, legible*)
(*boilerplate*)
↓

I have reviewed the test(s) you recently had done. The results are normal unless otherwise noted. For your own information, I have marked the test(s) that were performed.

___Complete Blood count	___Uric acid
___Kidney test	___Sed rate
___Liver test	___Potassium
___Thyroid test	___ANA (lupus test.)
_X_Prostate Specific Antigen (PSA)	___Electrocardiogram (EKG)
___Urinalysis	___Chest xray
___Blood sugar	___Alb/Creat Ratio

Hemoglobin A1C=___; This means your average blood sugar over the last 3 months was___.

If your cholesterol levels were checked, those are addressed in a separate letter.

Sincerely,

J Whistler RN (*scribbled, barely decipherable*)

for Dr Smathers (*scribbled but decipherable*)

Word/labtestresults/wmc
11/18/2002

CHAPTER 5

You perhaps think that this anecdote is atypical. My experience is otherwise. I can assure you that the above is not in the least an atypical or unusual report to a patient from a clinical laboratory. There is no indication that my relative's doctor ever saw or knew about the test results, since an intermediary (an RN) signed the report, and my relative didn't hear anything further from his doctor. He was left feeling both anxious and frustrated, because his doctor told him he had felt a small lump on his prostate gland by rectal examination. He called and asked me what I recommended that he do.

Further in this chapter I will present some ideas on how a laboratory director might choose to deliver a patient-oriented communication to an individual coming to the laboratory for medical service, and in so doing show you how important information was lost in this report of my relative's "normal" PSA in the illustration above.

An abnormal or marginal laboratory test report can, and should, be customized to meet the needs and concerns of the consumer. A report that simply provides information that "your test was normal" (or just numbers, as many laboratories do), may be readily understood by those acquainted with the limitations of laboratory tests, and their applicability to a specific medical question such as, "Is diabetes present?", or, "What is the likelihood of prostatic cancer?" But to those not so acquainted, raw numbers without a *frame of reference* (what is normal for the test) may be quite useless without an interpretation. In some instances misunderstanding of a test result's significance or implications may be both costly and dangerous.

Worse yet, lack of any numbers or no interpretation at all (as in the illustrative report above) smacks of an entirely inappropriate medical arrogance, with disregard for the needs and entitlement of a patient to know and understand the meanings, trends, implications and significance of every laboratory test result.

There are three categories of test report options that will meet the necessary information needs of most persons who order the test—healthcare provider or patient. A well run clinical laboratory can—and in my opinion should—offer such options.

A. Test results and normal values only, no medical interpretation.
B. Test results as in A, plus a differential diagnosis, urgency level, and limited medical interpretation.
C. Marginal and abnormal test results, including information from A and B, plus extensive medical consultative interpretation such as prognosis, important comments, and appropriate referral for follow-up care.

It is to be expected that laboratory charges for option A would likely be the least expensive; a test charge might be slightly higher for option B, and the charge for the extended report for option C could well be the highest, since medical advice, which entails knowledge, experience, and liability, is not included in the category A option, and only in limited amount in the category B option. Professional medical advice does have a monetary value in a free market system as in the US, and the charge for this value would be expected to be blended into the over-all charge for the test service.

Let's look at each one of these three options, A, B, and C in more detail, with examples of reports that might actually occur in a typical instance of a "normal" PSA test result": 4.4 ng/ml.

Test report option A

This option, the simplest, and most usual form of reporting test results provides numerical information only, with no further elaboration on the significance of the numbers. Such a basic report is appropriate if the test results are within the normal range—but only if it is a follow-up test when the supporting differential diagnosis, prognosis, appropriate follow-up, etc., have been supplied in a previous report. It is, however, far too limited in a report's potential for education and advice to a patient—or as a refresher or reminder to a healthcare provider!

Here is an example of a more enlightened and acceptable type of report many laboratories in the United States send out, in content, if not in similar format:

"Prostate Specific Antigen: 4.4 ng/ml.
Reference range:
up to age 69: < 4.5 ng/ml;
age 70 and over: < 6.6 ng/ml."

Test report option B

Option B would provide not only the test result information given in option A, but also would give a differential diagnosis *(see Chap. 4 to learn or refresh your memory about this)*. It would include some of the more important diseases or syndromes (groups of signs and *symptoms* that occur together and characterize a particular medical abnormality) that could be related to abnormal test results, presuming that the test results were out of the normal range; it could also include an urgency level, that is, whether the patient or the physician should take action immediately, or instead mull it over for awhile. Here is how this option might appear:

"Prostate Specific Antigen: 4.4 ng/ml.
Reference (normal) range:
up to age 69: < 4.5 ng/ml;
age 70 and over: < 6.6 ng/ml.
Differential diagnosis: None; test results are within
the reference range.
Urgency Level: None. Repeat the test in one year."

Test report option C

Option C for Prostate Specific Antigen goes beyond option B by giving not only a numerical test result, a differential diagnosis, and an urgency level, but also information on prognosis, factors influencing the test results that could skew or possibly invalidate them, and which medical specialist is appropriate for follow-up care. A report of this depth is essential when test results are abnormal or marginal. Here is an example of the information in a report for a "normal" PSA test result that is more detailed than just the numbers, differential diagnoses, and urgency level provided in option B:

"Prostate specific antigen (PSA): 4.4 ng/ml.
(borderline result)
Reference (normal) range:
up to age 69: < 4.5 ng/ml;
age 70 and over: < 6.6 ng/ml.
Differential diagnosis includes:
benign prostatic hypertrophy (BPH);
adenocarcinoma of the prostate gland; prostatitis.
Benign prostatic hypertrophy is a non-cancerous enlargement of the prostate gland that can cause a variety of symptoms such as frequency of urination or bladder infections; it is curable or controllable by surgery or medication.
Adenocarcinoma is a malignant tumor of the prostate gland that may be curable or treatable by surgery, radiation, or chemotherapy, or a combination of these.
Prostatitis is an inflammation of the prostate gland which may cause fever, pain, and urinary symptoms; it is usually curable or treatable with appropriate antibiotics.

Urgency level: Questionable: although the latest test result is still within the normal range, it is near an abnormal level; our records show that your PSA test results have been increasing over the years, and at an accelerating rate.

Factors influencing the test: Your PSA test result may be elevated if a digital rectal examination (DRE) was done shortly before the blood was taken for the test; if this is the case, it is suggested that the test be repeated.

Follow-up: Consult your physician; further testing and medical consultation with a urologist may be appropriate".

The three test report options described above are meant to show what a laboratory test report could—and should—include in this Information Age. Now that "medical imperialism is obsolete", many clinical pathologists believe that consumer demand for detailed reports on the results of their laboratory tests will push and prod medical directors of laboratories to meet a higher standard of reporting than now exists in many, if not most laboratories.

Perhaps now it would be appropriate to paraphrase Dr. Kassirer's quotation:

> *"The era of physicians' monopoly of laboratory test results*
> *is over. Laboratorian imperialism is obsolete."*

The following (fictitious) report is an example of how an informative test report might be designed to appear:

Illustration 2.

An example of a more appropriate report for a
Prostate Specific Antigen (PSA) test.
(all proper names are fictitious)

Wonderland Medical Center

CLINICAL LABORATORY REPORT
TEST RESULTS AND COMMENTARY

Name   : *John D oe*
Birthdate   : *09/21/47*
Address   : *234 Thermo Dr, Annapolis, IN*
Phone   : *(812) 673-4882*
Physician   : *Dr. Smathers*
Physician's Phone: *(812) 673-2677*

Specimen received: Date: *7/16/97* Time: *9:35 AM* By: *AJK*

Report Ready: Date: *7/16/97* Time: *11:33 AM*

Report option reqested: A___ B___ C___ √___

Report: Called___ Mailed___ FAXed___ Picked Up By: *Patient*

When: Date: *7/16/97* Time: *11:56 AM.*

TEST: Prostate Specific Antigen (PSA)

TEST RESULTS: 4.4 ng/ml. (see Comment below)

REFERENCE (NORMAL) RANGE:
up to age 60-69: < 4.5 ng/ml;
age 70 and over: < 6.6 ng/ml.

URGENCY LEVEL: Action:_____* Decision: _√_**

*   Action level: *a very abnormal test result that requires immediate action by the patient or healthcare provider.*

**   Decision level: *a test result above or below the reference (normal) range, or suggesting that a management action should be considered by a physician or the patient.*

A LIMITED DIFFERENTIAL DIAGNOSES:

benign prostatic hypertrophy, a non-cancerous enlargement of the prostate gland that can cause a variety of symptoms such as frequency of urination or bladder infections; it is curable or controllable by surgery or medication;
adenocarcinoma of the prostate gland, a malignant tumor of the prostate gland that may be curable or treatable, often causing symptoms as in benign prostatic hypertrophy, but often can be asymptomatic;
prostatitis, an inflammation of the prostate gland which may cause fever, pain, and urinary symptoms; it is curable or treatable.

POSSIBLE INTERFERENCES with the PSA test: Recent digital examination of the prostate gland through the rectum may elevate the PSA.

COMMENT: Although the test result is within the normal range for your age, your file in this laboratory indicates a persistent upward and accelerating trend in your PSA test results:

2/12/94: 2.5 ng/mL
3/17/95: 2.9 ng/mL (0.4 ng/mL increase)
1/31/96: 3.5 ng/mL (0.6 ng/mL increase)
12/7/97: 4.4 ng/mL. (0.9 ng/mL increase).

While this trend is not specifically diagnostic, it suggests that a reason for these increases over time should be sought by your physician; it could indicate a localized cancer of the prostate gland at a time when it is curable.

FOLLOW-UP: Consult your physician for advice about cost-effective further testing, and advice about physician specialists to contact for follow-up, e.g., urologist, oncologist, geriatrician.

Rule of thumb: If the test result does not conform with your or your physician's clinical impression, the test should be repeated!

(*signature or initials*)
Martin J. Goodspeed, M.D., FASCP, FCAP
Laboratory Director

It is clear that options A and B failed to give important information, the upward and accelerating trend of the patient's test results over the years. This critical information is disclosed and discussed in option C. The implications for the health and well-being of the fictitious "John Doe"—as well as many real patients—should be obvious to laboratory directors and clinical pathologists who are not presenting test data in a format that displays significant trends in test results over time.

Computer storage of data on a patient's previous tests, and setting up macros and templates on a word processor to provide useful consultative information to the patient and the patient's healthcare provider is not a daunting task for the clinical pathologist. This has been pointed out to clinical pathologists in my medical text, *Actions and Decisions: Concise Consultations for the Clinical Pathologist,* published by the ASCP Press of the American Society of Clinical Pathologists.

CHAPTER 6

Numbers and Normal Ranges

In the United States the numbers used in expressing test results are based on the metric system. These numbers are referred to as "customary" or "conventional" units, but they are only customary or conventional in the United States and a very few other countries around the globe. The units of weight are expressed as *grams (g), milligrams (mg), nanograms (ng)*, or *picograms (pg)*, and units of volume as *liters (L), deciliters (dL)*, or *milliliters (ml)*, and many of the tests in this section are expressed *per deciliter (/dL)*.

More commonly used, based on gram-molecular weights (as explained to you in your high school chemistry course, remember?) and agreed upon by most medical scientists outside the United States as being more appropriate, are different units of data expression; these are referred to as (going from larger to smaller) *mols* or fractions of mols, e.g., *millimols (mmol), micromols (mmol), nanomols (nmol), picomols (pmol)*, etc., and expressed *per liter (/L)*. *Systeme Internationale d'Unites (SI)* are used in expressing test result data in much of the world's scientific literature.

In Part III, Interpretations, numbers for both normal (reference) ranges and examples of test results are expressed in customary units for U.S. consumers and healthcare workers, but also in *SI* units for the convenience of those living outside the U.S.

Here is a short refresher about fluid volumes and weights as used in the expression of medical laboratory test results:

fluids:
> a *liter* (L), equals very close to a quart of fluid
> a *deciliter* (dL, also dl) is one tenth of a liter
> a *milliliter* (mL, also, ml) is one one-thousandth of a liter;

weights (metric, conventional in US):
> a *kilogram* (kg) equals very close to 2.20 U.S. lb.
> a *gram* (g) equals one thousandth of a kilogram
> a *milligram* (mg) is one thousandth of a gram.
> a *microgram* (mg) is one millionth of a gram
> a *nanogram* (ηg) is one billionth of a gram
> a *picogram* (ρg) is one trillionth of a gram

weights (molecular, SI):
> a *mol* (mol) is the gram-molecular weight of a substance
> a *millimol* (mmol) is one thousandth of a mol
> a *micromol* (mmol) is one millionth of a mol
> a *nanomol* (ηmol) is one billionth of a mol
> a *picomol* (ρmol) is one trillionth of a mol

Here is an example (using the two means of expression, customary and *SI*) that gives identical information for the same amount of glucose in a blood sample:

> *using the customary or conventional system:*
> glucose: 100 mg/dL
> *using the SI system:*
> glucose: 5.6 mmol/L,
> thus,
> 100 mg/dL of glucose is the same as 5.6 mmol/L of glucose.

Now that you have this background, the reference (normal) range values in both systems for the tests in Table 4 and in Part III Interpretations should be understandable. Many of the test normals—those that are not expressed in numbers (e.g., Positive, Negative, WNL, ABO and Rh blood groups, etc.)—will be the same in both systems. Presently, readers in the U.S. need not bother with SI units when reviewing their test results, since few U.S. laboratories use this system—unfortunately, but for reasons not to be belabored here.

Table 4

Normal Values
Some examples of Customary and *SI* Unit Values

Laboratory Test	Customary Values	Systeme Internationale
Activated partial thromboplastin time	25-39 seconds	25-39 seconds
Bilirubin, conjugated (direct)	= or < 0.4 mg/dL	= or < 7.0 mmol/L
Blood alcohol	< 10 mg/dL	< 10 mmol/L
Blood sugar, random:	60-115 mg/dL	3.3 - 6.4 mmol/L
borderline normal:	116-125mg/dL	6.4 -6.9 mmol/L
Blood type and group	(not applicable in either system: descriptive data)	
Blood urea nitrogen (BUN)	5 - 20 mg/dL	1.8 - 7.1 mmol/L

CHAPTER 7

Preparation for Laboratory Tests

I n general, it is best to enquire of the laboratory before going for testing to make sure that there are no special requirements for preparation for the tests you are about to have performed, and if there are specific requirements, to adhere to these carefully to avoid invalid test results, and therefore a waste of your (or someone's) money. Most tests do not require special preparation, but check this out before arriving for testing at the laboratory that will be doing the test. A few frequently performed tests included in Part III do require some preparation and are mentioned here:

Most laboratory tests that don't mention "Fasting" in their names do not require any special preparation. However, a few tests, like the Fasting Blood Sugar and the Glucose Tolerance (which doesn't mention fasting in the title) do require special preparation, and the laboratory will provide that information at your request, prior to your arrival for testing. Some panels, such as Cardiac Risk include a test (e.g., Apo A and B, triglyderides) that should be done on a fasting specimen; often this is mistakenly or intentionally overlooked.

Stool examination for Occult Blood does require quite a rigorous adherence to diet for several days before and during collection of the specimen. False-positives may be the result of failure to observe these instructions, and the consequences involve extensive follow-up testings which can be as expensive as they may be unpleasant.

Sputum Cytology specimens are best collected *after deep coughing* (really trying to cough hard from deep down in the chest) early in the morning, because the richest accumulation of cells of diagnostic quality is to be found in this type of sputum sample.

Semen analysis must be performed on a clean, fresh, warm specimen, best collected at the laboratory facility by masturbation privately in the laboratory toilet facilities.

Vitamin B_{12} blood specimens require testing after refraining from taking multivitamins for at least a week, and may only be valid when a specimen is collected several weeks after the last B_{12} injection.

A Papanicalou Cytology Smear for screening for cancer of the cervix, endometrium and vagina must be obtained without prior douching; douching would likely remove most or all of the cells necessary for diagnosis in the smear. Also, nothing should be inserted in the vagina for 48 hours prior to obtaining the smear specimen.

Blood alcohol tests for legal purposes should be done as soon as possible after the suspicion of intoxication has been raised.

Remember, it is always wise to contact the receptionist at the laboratory of your choice beforehand to be certain that there are no special preparations you need to undertake before going to the laboratory for *any* testing.

CHAPTER 8

Direct Access Testing

F inding a clinical laboratory that is reputable and dependable is not hard. Almost all hospital and commercial laboratories are accredited by either the College of American Pathologist's Inspection and Accreditation Program (CAP I&A), the Joint Commission on Accreditation of Hospitals Organization (JCAHO), or one or several state and federal agencies. Laboratories that do not meet the stringent criteria for accreditation, licensing, or certification do not stay in business very long. So it is very likely that in the United States at least, any hospital or commercial clinical medical laboratory will be a reliable and dependable source of medical data. Of course problems can crop up between inspections which might allow a laboratory to slip below standards, but these will presumably become apparent at the next inspection. In the interim, no laboratory wishes to face the possibility of litigation because of sub-standard performance and resultant serious medical malpractice, so there is a strong incentive to maintain high quality laboratory services.

Private clinical laboratories in physician's offices do not always undergo such rigid scrutiny by professional organizations such as the College of American Pathologists, or by state and federal agencies, although some may request such inspection to assure a high level of quality. Thus, while many office laboratories may provide high quality laboratory test results, in some, test performance and reliability may be questionable. *Caveat emptor!*

How does one go about getting a laboratory test without using a physician as an intermediary? The answer is Direct Access Testing (DAT).

Although the concept of DAT is sound, and many laboratory directors believe in it, the truth is that this belief is far from universal. Many laboratories will accept a request for service from a concerned citizen without the mediation of a physician or a physician's assistant, but many will not. Why is this, in the age of consumerism?

Well, as Tevye says in *Fiddler on the Roof:* "Tradition! Tra-di-tion!" Many laboratories have always done it the traditional way, only testing when a *doctor* has ordered it. And there may be good reasons for that, not necessarily obvious to the person walking into a laboratory with a test request on his or her mind. Let's look at some of these reasons and some of the problems.

Medical laboratories include public health laboratories, research laboratories, and clinical laboratories. The latter are those that serve the public for medical diagnostic purposes. Clinical laboratories are basically of three types: the physician's office or clinic laboratory; the hospital laboratory; and the commercial laboratory. DAT availability is determined by the attitudes of the owners and managers of clinical laboratories. These attitudes may vary considerably, so let's examine these attitudes and the reasons behind them.

The Physician Office or Clinic Laboratory

This laboratory is owned by a physician, a group of physicians, a clinic, or a health maintenance organization (HMO). The owner(s) would like their patients to have tests that only *they* feel are clinically necessary. In addition, unless they restrict testing to patients in their own practices, they have to undergo rigorous federal and state regulation of the quality and extent of testing that is done in their laboratory. Also, the physicians may see some economic virtue in seeing the patient both before and after the test is done. (Only the most cynical, of course, could suspect that the addition of one or two office visit charges to the laboratory bill might be a consideration; no one wants to be suspicious of the motives of the person who may be making life and death decisions now or in the future, for if we suspect him, her, or them in little things, what confidence would we have when the big things come along?).

Also, where the physician is a gatekeeper working in a managed care facility and his or her income may be enhanced by rigorously containing expenses, laboratory testing may be somewhat limited in general. It is clear that for any or all of the above reasons, direct access testing is unlikely at this type of laboratory.

The Hospital Laboratory

The hospital laboratory is owned and operated by the hospital; sometimes, particularly in isolated or rural areas the hospital is the only source of laboratory services available. These laboratories undergo rigorous inspection by national accrediting organizations before they receive accreditation, something necessary if they are to be reimbursed for services to Medicare and Medicaid patients—a big part of their business (yes, a hospital *is* a business). The hospital laboratory must have a laboratory director (usually a pathologist) who may favor DAT, but he or she may not be making policy. The hospital's trustees may think direct access testing is too new or too risky, or as sometimes happens, they just don't understand the concept.

And if the hospital administrator happens not to want to add any new troubles to existing woes, he or she may advise the trustees not to touch it. The situation is often different in more populated areas where several hospitals serve the town or city and the competition has become intense for patients or patient panels and the associated revenues. Here, DAT may be more readily available.

Commercial Laboratories and Reference Laboratories

Commercial laboratories, those not related to a medical facility, often serve as backup for hospitals and physician office laboratories because of their ability to provide testing not feasible or possible at these smaller facilities. They are in a strong position to accommodate the public with DAT because of their greater resource bases in capital, equipment, and personnel. It is likely that these accredited laboratories will be found to be in the forefront of offering DAT, primarily because of their profit-based orientation. Hospital laboratories, in competition with these commercial and reference laboratories likely may be encouraged or forced to follow this lead, especially if they have a laboratory director who favors DAT and a CEO whose hospital needs the money.

Other Thoughts

But our society is complex, and there are some realities consumers should know about. Perhaps highest on the list of resistance to DAT has to do with legal liability, a subject lurking in the back of the physician's mind every day of practice (refer to the frontispiece of this book!). Many physicians, including some pathologist laboratory directors, avoid DAT because they fear this liability. They may feel that no matter how many disclaimers they may print on the report forms about freedom from responsibility should something untoward happen as a result of a patient's actions after receiving a test report, the risk cannot be totally obviated. Sometimes their attorneys or their insurance carriers feel the same way, and have advised the hospital or the laboratory director to avoid DAT. One successful lawsuit by a customer (we can hardly use the term *patient* in DAT unless a doctor is somehow involved, and he or she may not be) can wipe out any profit for the laboratory, now, or perhaps into the distant future if a settlement is big enough.

Less important, but often the case, the lack of a system for handling this different aspect of laboratory service may act as a deterrent to a decision to provide DAT. How does one collect the money? And when? Up front, or after the test report is received? Use credit cards? How about third-party payer hassles? Questions like this weigh heavily on the side of not rocking the boat, not doing something new and untried that might bring troubles far beyond the hoped for benefits to the provider of the service.

Also, some physicians may be concerned (realistically in some cases) that the patient will use the test results without an understanding of their significance. A proper laboratory report (you've read about this in *Chapter 5, What You Should Expect in a Laboratory Test Report*) should provide the patient with suggestions regarding what to do with the information. But patient compliance with the doctor's advice and instructions is a similar problem; trust is always necessary on each side of the doctor-patient relationship.

DAT and Wellness

And so we come to DAT and its relationship to wellness. As the concept of preventive healthcare gains momentum, the citizenry is becoming more aware of what this means in practical terms to them. More concern with fitness, weight control, avoidance of abusive substances such as tobacco and alcohol, and the use of sunscreens on the skin are all evidence of this. A natural outgrowth of this interest in preserving health is the desire for knowledge of what is going on inside the body as well as what can be seen in the mirror or felt with the fingers. This is just the thing that clinical laboratory tests can do: relieve worries about things that may be lurking within and that can be neither seen nor felt from the outside.

Tests for bleeding in the stomach or intestines, diabetes, excess lipids and lipoproteins in the blood, anemia, gout, pregnancy, and many other concerns are now quite easily performed with modern laboratory techniques. There need no longer be great ceremony or mystery involved with getting tests done to uncover hidden disease. Whether in the name of fitness, early detection of disease, relief of worry, or simply curiosity, if concerned individuals choose to use their resources to acquire information about their own bodies, there is no reason to deny this freedom to them. In the author's opinion DAT should be available to any who want it and are willing to pay for it. Indeed, in the EU there are already free-standing commercial laboratories dedicated to DAT available to the public.

It seems that DAT may well be a reality whose time has come. Physicians who are now skeptical may eventually come to realize that DAT is not a fad, that it is here to stay. And if their patient's health is their real concern it makes sense to develop and encourage the patient's responsibility for his or her own well-being by using all resources available to each of them.

CHAPTER 8

CHAPTER 9

Interpretation Formats, Tests for Symptoms

and Worries, and Normal Values for Tests

The Interpretations in following Part III are presented in formats that assume that each of the tests has been done on a fictitious patient and a hypothetical result has been obtained. Usually that result is presented in these examples as abnormal, and more often than not at an Action ("panic") level of urgency. The author's intent in doing this is to present a worst-possible situation so that should a reader's personal test result ever come back at an Action level of urgency he or she will be motivated to make the proper response: to call or see a physician at once.

The reader is reminded that most test results fall within the normal range, or perhaps just a little outside of the normal range for the test. As mentioned in *Chapter 3*, there is no need to be unduly distressed just because a Decision level report is received, but discussion about the meaning of the test result with a physician or other knowledgeable health care provider is surely the best approach. Decision level results should never be dismissed as unimportant. The best move is to have the test done again for confirmation, and to have both test results reviewed by the professional who is being consulted for advice. Let me give you an anecdotal personal experience to emphasize this.

Doctors too—even pathologists—are mortal, and I recently had a brief visit to the Emergency Room in a local hospital. Blood was drawn from a vein in my arm by a nurse with a less-than-desirable aptitude for the task. She used a too-large needle and managed to puncture my vein in such a way that blood leaked out into the surrounding tissues, and the blood she obtained was also slightly diluted with the interstitial tissue fluid surrounding the vein. The result was a hemoglobin value that was a substantial amount lower than the normal range for a male's hemoglobin, and lower than the hemoglobin test that had been done five months before at my annual health examination. This was noted by the doctor looking after me, and we discussed whether perhaps a colonoscopy was needed.

Of course this raised my anxiety level substantially, because when there is such a drop in hemoglobin after a short interval without other symptoms, doctors know that a common cause is internal bleeding from cancer of the colon. However, my stool examination for occult blood was reassuringly negative at the time of my prior health examination. So I went to the laboratory and had my blood tested again. This time the blood was taken from my vein expertly by the laboratory's phlebotomist, using the proper size needle. When the test result was available a short time later my hemoglobin was found to be back within the normal range, and of course my anxiety level decreased considerably.

There are several lessons to be learned here, but probably the most important is that if laboratory tests are abnormal and don't fit with other information your doctor has, it is worthwhile to have the abnormal results rechecked. In my case had this testing not been repeated, an expensive cascade of unnecessary events probably would have followed.

It must be remembered that there are many prescribed, as well as over-the-counter medications that interfere with laboratory test results. Unfortunately many healthcare providers overlook these drug interferences with laboratory tests because of failure to ask the patient if he or she was taking medications, or because of a lack of knowledge about possible influences these medications might have on the test results. So it is imperative that the person going to the laboratory for testing advise the laboratorians of any drugs he or she is taking. If no one asks about this, the information should be volunteered. The information can make a great difference in how the test results are interpreted, and what might follow.

It must be emphasized that the laboratory tests included in this book are usually only indicators of, or adjuncts to, the diagnosis of disease. Diagnosis in almost all instances must be part of a thorough and thoughtful investigation of a patient's symptoms, medical history, physical signs, laboratory tests, as well as other investigative procedures by a physician.

For example, a patient suffering from depression might have a thyroid stimulating hormone (TSH) test performed that indicates hypothyroidism, but clinical depression is only occasionally the result of hypothyroidism; many other causes exist as well for this common problem. Conversely, a normal TSH test result certainly does not establish the absence of clinical depression. The laboratory test is just a piece of the diagnostic puzzle.

Another important warning is that negative test results do not assure that a problem does not exist. Tests for sexually transmitted diseases (STD) are notoriously unreliable in guaranteeing that a problem doesn't exist. Some studies have shown that urethral or vaginal cultures may miss uncovering STD such as gonorrhea in as many as 70% of the individuals tested when only conventional test procedures are used. Examples of important *pathogenic* (disease-causing) infectious agents that could be missed by such cultures are *herpes virus* and *papilloma virus*, because these infections require special culture techniques to discover them.

And remember that if your worries persist repetition of a test at reasonable periodic intervals may provide information that a trend is taking place, something that a single test result cannot show. Trends are important in the development of chronic diseases such as anemia, osteoporosis, diabetes, prostatic cancer, or AIDS (*see Chapter 5, Test report option C*). Sad to say, many physicians are unaware of trends in their patients' test results because of the way laboratory test data are filed in their patient's clinical records. If you find this to be the case, you can bring a trend to your physician's attention with test data you have compiled yourself as a result of direct access testing and by keeping your own file of all laboratory test results you have received, especially if the tests have been done at one or more different laboratories. Fortunately, most up-to-date clinical laboratories have computer programs that compile and report prior test results in such a manner that it will show trends over time.

Do not lightly disregard laboratory reports that indicate that a test result is "H" (high), or "L" (low). While most data so designated are not causes for panic, it is important to find out their significance. This is best done by consulting a physician who is knowledgeable about your health history and who will give either reassurance that the abnormality is of no significance, or initiate actions such as ordering a repetition of the test that will help identify the cause of the test result aberration.

And remember that you are entitled to get a complete report of test results from your health care provider, not just some numbers that you don't understand, or a report that "your tests all came out okay".

Here is a quote from a recent *Consumer Reports on Health* worthy of note:

> "No news is not always good news when it comes to medical tests. Sometimes it means health professionals have failed to process or communicate

test results. Ask your doctor when you can expect to hear about test results, and follow up if you're not contacted."

That's a warning to take to heart.

Table 5

Where to Find Appropriate Tests for Typical Symptoms or Worries

SYMPTOM OR WORRY	AN APPROPRIATE TEST	CHAPTER
Infection of skin, or subcutaneous tissue with fever (e.g., "stepped on a rusty nail")	Wound and/or Blood Culture	11
Feel lousy but no specific symptoms	C-Reactive Protein (CPR); Monospot: CBC; ESR	11, 13
Diarrhea and cramps: drank brook water while hiking	Stool for Giardia	11
Yellow eyeballs and/or yellow skin	Liver Panel	11
Think I might have "mono".	Heterophil Antibody; Monospot™	11
Exposed to HIV infection	HIV1/HIV2	11
Tick bite and joints ache	Lyme Disease Serology	11
Persistent diarrhea since trip outside the U.S.	Ova and Parasites in Stool; Stool Culture	11
Been exposed sexually without protection	HIV1/HIV2; RPR Serology; Urethral Culture; Vaginal Culture	11
Baby or child has a sore throat and fever	Streptococcus ("Strep") Screen	11
Bad sore throat	Throat Culture; Monospot™	11
Discharge from penis	Urethral Culture; RPR for Syphilis	11
Burning on urination	Urine Culture; Urinalysis with micro (UA)	11

Vaginal discharge	Vaginal Culture; Pap smear	11
Worry about cholesterol	Cholesterol; Cardiac Risk	12
Anemia; tired all the time; persistent heavy menstrual periods	Complete Blood Count (CBC); Serum Iron	15
My baby eats everything and we live in an old house with lead	Serum Lead	12
Worry about colon cancer; blood in my stool (or on toilet	Hemoccultă	14
Haven't had a Pap test annually; vaginal bleeding	Papanicalou Cytologic Test ("Pap Smear")	12
Prostate cancer; urinary difficulties	Prostate Specific Antigen	12; 22
Diabetes; thirsty all the time and urinate a lot; lost weight	Random or Fasting Blood Sugar (FBS)	15
Tired all the time; no pep; hair feels dry	Thyroid Stimulating Hormone (TSH); Vitamin B 12	12
Bruise easily and taking blood-thinner medicine	Activated Partial Thromboplastin Time (APTT); Prothrombin time (PT)	13
Bulemia and worry about anemia because of it	Complete Blood Count (CBC); Serum Iron (SI)	13
Bruise easily	Complete Blood Count	13
Is my blood-thinner (Warfarin) dose right?	Prothrombin Time	13, 24
My face is very ruddy and it's not sunburn or windburn	Complete Blood Count (CBC)	13
Swollen glands (lymph nodes) armpits/ groin/ behind jaw	Complete Blood Count; Monospot™	11; 13
Have been treated for cancer of the colon and worried it's	Carcinoembryonic Antigen (CEA); Liver Panel	14, 15
What does "ERA-PRA" in my pathology report mean?	Estrogen and Progesterone Receptor Assay (ERA-PRA)	10
Smoker with bloody sputum and/or cough	Sputum Cytology	14
Aching joints and rash on my cheeks	Arthritis Panel; Anti-DNA; Anti-Nuclear Antibody (ANA)	15
HIV positive and wonder if my treatment is helping	CD4/CD8 Lymphocyte Count and Ratio	15

CHAPTER 9

Does my child have Cystic Fibrosis? It's in my family.	Chloride Sweat Test; Cystic Fibrosis DNA Content	15
Feel faint and worry about low blood sugar	Glucose Tolerance Test (GTT)	15
Recurring belly pains	*Helicobacter pylori* Serologic Test	15
I'm diabetic and wonder if my blood sugar is under control	Hemoglobin A1c	15
Have diabetes; family history of kidney disease	Kidney Panel	15
Have arthritis and worry about "Lupus"	LE Cell Test	15
Worry about osteoporosis	Osteocalcin	15
Stiff and/or swollen joints	Rheumatoid Factor (RF); Uric Acid	15
I'm hyper and jittery ; can't sleep at night	Thyroxine (T4)	15
Swollen and red big toe	Uric Acid	15
Chest pain and heart attack	CK-MB; Troponin	16
Afraid of a heart attack; I'm overweight and a smoker	Cardiac Risk Assessment	16
Flunked the alcohol breath test; lawyer says I need a blood	Blood Alcohol	18
I *know* I'm not the father of my ex-girl friend's baby	Paternity Test Panel	18
Lost interest in sex	Testosterone	19
Wonder whether I'm going through menopause or pregnant	Menopause Panel; Beta subunit Human Chorionic Gonadotropin (HCG)	20
Is my unborn baby going to be okay?	Alpha1 fetoprotein; Amniocentesis	22
Missed my period; am I pregnant?	Beta subunit Human Chorionic Gonadotropin (HCG)	21
Pregnancy	Folic Acid	21
Pregnant with a history of miscarriages	Progesterone	21
Vasectomy check	Semen Analysis, including Sperm Count	21

CHAPTER 9

Prostate cancer spread	Prostate Acid Phosphatase	22
Prostate needle biopsy pathology report grading (Gleason grade)	Prostate Needle Biopsy grading	10; 22
What screening tests should my kids have?	Serun Lead; Cholesterol; Random Blood Sugar; Sexually Transmited	12; 23
Ears ringing: toxic dose of my Aspirin?	Aspirin	24
Heart rate very slow: does my heart medicine need checking?	Digoxin	24
Toxic dose of my Dilantin?	Phenytoin (Dilantin)	24
Muscles twitching, and blurred vision: toxic dose of Lithium?	Lithium	24
Nose bleeds: toxic dose of my Heparin?	Activated Partial Thromboplastin Time (APTT)	13; 24
Nose bleeds: toxic dose of my Warfarin?	Prothrombin Time	13; 24
Wheezing again; right dose of Theophylline?	Theophylline	24
Haven't had a health check-up in quite a while.	Panel: Annual Check-up	12; 17

Table 6

Normal Values for Tests

LABORATORY TEST	CONVENTIONAL NORMAL VALUES	SYSTEME INTERNATIONALE NORMAL VALUES
Activated partial thromb -oplastin	25 - 39 seconds	25 - 39 seconds
Alanine aminotrans-ferase (ALT)	varies by test method (see Chapter 11, Liver Panel)	
Alkaline phosphatase	varies by test method (see Chapter 11, Liver Panel)	

Alphafeto-protein	< 10 mg/ml	
Anti-DNA (Anti-dsDNA)	less than 70 units	
Antiglobulin	negative*	
Anti-nuclear antibody (ANA)	negative fluorescence	
Apoliporotein A and B	(see *Chapter 16, Cardiac Risk Panel*)	
Arthritis panel	(*see Chapter 15 for RF, LE cells, Uric Acid*)	
Aspartate aminotrans-ferase (AST)	varies by test method (*see Chapter 11, Liver Panel*)	
Aspirin	negative*; (see Interpretation for therapeutic levels)	
Bilirubin, conjugated (direct)	= or < 0.4 mg/dL	= or < 7.0 mmol/L
Blood alcohol	< 10 mg/dL	< 10 mmol/L
Blood count, complete (CBC)	varies by sex and age; (*see: Chapter 13, #3*)	
Blood culture	no growth	
Blood lead	less than 10 ug/dL	
Blood sugar, fasting and random:	60 - 115 mg/dL 60 - 115 mg/dL "borderline normal": 116 -125 mg/dL	3.3 - 6.4 mmol/L 3.3 - 6.4 mmol/L 6.4 - 6.9 mmol/L
Blood type and group	(not applicable)	
Blood urea nitrogen (BUN)	5 - 20 mg/dL	1.8 - 7.1 mmol/L

Carcino-embryonic antigen	non-smoker: < 2.5 ng/mL; smoker: < 5.0 ng/mL	non smoker: < 2.5 mg/L; smoker: < 5.0 mg/L
Cardiac Risk assessment	(see Chapter 16, Cardiac Risk Panel)	
CD4/CD8 lymphocyte ratio	(see Chapter 15, Chronic Disease Tests)	
Chloride sweat test	negative*	
Cholesterol, total	varies with age	
Chorionic gonadotrpin	> 50 IU/L	> 50 IU/L
Creatine phosphokinase (CK)	males: 50 - 200 U/L females: 40 - 150 U/L	same same
Creatine phosphokinase CK-MB fraction	< 6% of CK	same
Cobalamin (Vitamin B12)	(approximate): 100 -250 rg/ml	(approximate): 74 - 185 rmol/L
Complete blood count (CBC)	(see Chapter 13: Hb, Hct, RBC, WBC, Platelets, Smear review)	
C-reactive protein (CRP)	less than 8 mg/dL	less tha 80 mg/L
Cystic fibrosis (CF) DNA content	0-40 mmol/L (usual range; many laboratories give interpretive report)	0-40 mmol/L (usual range; many laboratories give interpretive report)
Creatinine	0.3 - 1.2 mg/dL	26.5 - 106 mmol/L
Creatinine clearance	75 - 125 mL/minute	
Digoxin	negative*; therapeutic range: 0.5 - 2.8 ng/mL	0.6 - 3.6 mmol/L
Dilantin (Phenytoin)	negative*; (see Chapter 21 for therapeutic levels)	

CHAPTER 9

Estrogens	(see Chapter 20, Menopause Tests)	
Estrogen and progesterone receptor assay (ERA - PRA)	Positive or Strongly Positive	
Fasting blood sugar	60 -115 mg/dL	3.3 - 6.4 mmol/L
Ferritin	12 - 263 ng/mL	12 - 263 mg/L
Folic acid	> 2 ng/ml	> 5nmol/L
Gamma glutamyl transferase	varies by test method (see Chapter 11, #8, #9, Liver Panels)	
Giardia lamblia in stool	negative*; or "no Giardia present"	
Glucose tolerance test (GTT)	(see Chapter 15, Chronic Disease)	
Hepatitis panel	(see Chapter 11, Liver Panel)	
HDL cholesterol	(see Chapter 12, Cholesterol)	
Cholesterol: TC:HDLC ratio	(see Chapter 16, Cardiac Risk)	
Helicobacter	negative*	
pylori serologic test		
Hematocrit	female: 38 - 44% male: 43 - 49%	
Hemoglobin	female: 12.7-14.7 gm/dL male: 14.7 - 16.7 gm/dL	
Hemoglobin A1c	4% - 6.5%	4% -6.5%

Hemoglobin-opathies	*(see Chapter 13, #5, Anemia, etc.)*	
Heparin	*(see Chapter 24, #1, APTT)*	
Hepatitis panel	*(see Chapter 11, #8, #9 Liver Function)*	
Heterophile antibody	negative*	
HIV1/HIV2 serology	negative*	
Homocysteine (Urinary cystine)	40-60 mg cystine/g of creatinine *(see Chapter 16, Cardiac Risk Assesment)*	
Iron, serum	60 - 160 mg/dL	11 - 29 mmol/L
Infectious mononucleosis ("Mono" test)	negative*	
Kidney panel	*(see Chapter 15, component tests)*	
Kidney stones	(not applicable)	
Lactic dehydrog'nase	< 200 units/L	< 96 IU/L
LDL cholesterol	*(see Chapter 16, Heart Disease Tests)*	
LE cell	negative*	
Lead (serum)	< 10 mg/dL	
Libido	*(see Chapter 18, Testosterone for males and females)*	
Lithium	0.0 mEq/L	0.0 mmol/L

Liver panel	(*see Chapter 11, #8, #9 Liver Disease component tests*)	
Lupus erythematosus (LE)	negative*	
Lyme Disease serology	negative*	
Occult blood in stool ("Hemoccult")	negative*	
Osteocalcin pre- menopausal: post- menopausal:	0.4 - 0.8 ng/mL 3.0 -12.0 ng/ml	0.4 - 8.0 mg/L
Ova and parasites in stool	negative*	3.0 -12.0 mg/L
Papanicalou smear	normal, or negative* for malignant cells	
Papanicalou smear maturation index	(*see Chapter 14, Cancer Screening Tests*)	
Paternity	(not applicable)	
Phenytoin	negative*; (*see Chapter 24 for therapeutic level*)	
Platelet count (CBC)	150 -450,000/cu mm	150 - 450, x 10^9/L
Pregnancy test	negative*	
Prenatal screen	(*see Chapter 21, ABO, D, Du, AHG*)	
Prostate specific antigen	Age-related; upper threshholds: 40's: 2.5 ng/ml 50's : 3.5 ng/ml 60's: 4.0 ng/ml 70+: < 4.5 ng/ml	

Prothrombin time	10 - 13 seconds	10 - 13 seconds
Random blood sugar	60 - 115 mg/dL; "borderline" normal: 116 - 125mg/dL	3.3 - 6.4 mmol/L 6.4 - 6.9 mmol/L
Rapid Plasmin Reagin (RPR)	negative*	
Red blood cell count (RBC)	female: $3.5 - 5.0 \times 10^{6}$/cu mm male: $4.3 - 5.9 \times 10^{6}$/cu mm	$3.5 - 5.0 \times 10^{12}$/L $4.3 - 5.9 \times 10^{12}$/L
Rheumatoid factor	negative*	
Salicylate	(see Chapter 24, Aspirin)	
Semen analysis	(see Chapter 21, Pregnancy and Infertility)	
Sexually transmitted diseases	(see: Chapter 23, HIV1/HIV2, Urethral culture, Vaginal culture, RPR for syphilis)	
Smear review (blood smear)	Segs: 51 +/- 15% Bands: 8 +/- 3% Lymphs: 34 +/- 10% Monos: 4% Eos: 2 +/- 1% Basos: 0.5& Platelets: WNL*	
Sputum cytology	negative* for malignant cells	
Strep screen	negative* for streptococci	
Stool culture	normal flora	
Testosterone	(see Chapter 19, Libido)	
Theophylline	negative*	

CHAPTER 9

Throat culture	negative* for pathogens	
Thyroid stimulating hormone (TSH)	0.4 - 4.2 mIU/L	0.4 - 4.2 mIU/L
Thyroxine	5.8 - 11.0 mg/dL	75 - 142 nmol/L
Transferrin (TIBC)	200 - 380 mg/dL	2.0 - 3.8 g/L
Transferrin Saturation	20 - 50 %	20 - 50%
Triglycerides (TG)	(see *Chapter 16, Cardiac Risk Assessment*)	
Troponin	< 0.35 ng/mL	
Urethral culture	negative*; no growth	
Uric acid	2.0 - 7.0 mg/dL	120 - 420 umol/L
Urine culture	less than 1000 CFU or negative*	
Urinalysis with micro	normal* (*see Chapter 12, Annual Check-Up Screening Tests*)	
Urine culture	negative*	
Vaginal culture	normal flora	
Warfarin (Dicumarol)	(*see Chapter 24, Prothrombin Time*)	
White blood cell count	3,200 -9,800/cu mm	3.2 - 9.8x 10^9/L

*   "negative" and "within normal limits" ("WNL") are synonymous with "normal".

II

Understanding Your Surgical Biopsy Report

FOREWORD

T his section will help you understand the sometimes strange or confusing terms used by pathologists in their surgical pathology reports and their meaning in relation to your health. It will also help you understand whether the lesion that has been removed from your body is due to infection, or if it represents a benign or malignant tumor. The treatment, if any is necessary, to cure, control or alleviate the lesion described and diagnosed by the pathologist will be based on this diagnosis and its implications. Therefore it is important that you understand completely what this means for your health and future well-being. You may well have to make a choice based on your understanding of the meaning of the report. Sometimes this may be quite difficult, but you are ultimately the one responsible for the decision about which course of further action your physician or surgeon should take in your behalf.

CHAPTER 10

Your Surgical Pathology Biopsy Report

W hen a surgeon or a physician removes a piece of tissue from your body, the tissue becomes a *tissue specimen* that must be examined by a *pathologist*. A pathologist is a physician who has undergone lengthy training in the specialty of *pathology*. Pathology is defined as the study of disease. It is a medical specialty, one of many specialties in the field of medicine and surgery. A *board certified pathologist* is a physician who has passed examination and scrutiny by the American Board of Pathology (ABP). The ABP is a group of distinguished and experienced peers in the specialty who have established qualifications and standards of education, residency training, experience, and competence necessary for certification. To become board certified, a candidate must pass rigorous training for four years followed by written and practical examinations.

When the tissue specimen from a biopsy or organ removal during surgery is received in the laboratory, the pathologist carefully examines the entire specimen, and then takes one or more representative portions for further examination under the microscope. In a day or so, the pathologist makes a written report, a *surgical pathology report*, that gives the diagnosis. This is sent to the patient's surgeon or physician.

The pathologist's examination always takes place, whether the biopsy is done in a doctor's office, a clinic, an emergency room, or the operating room in a hospital. If tissue removed is not so examined, there is the possibility of a wrong or an unsuspected diagnosis with perhaps unfortunate consequences. Every physician is aware of this—as is the legal profession. A copy of the pathologist's report should be available to any patient who requests it. It should be read by the patient in the presence of the surgeon, who should then and there help the patient comprehend the meaning of the report in terms the patient can understand.

Illustration 3.

A fictitious Surgical Pathology report of a mastectomy specimen examination and pathologic diagnosis
(all proper names are fictitious)

Wonderland Medical Center
Department of Pathology

Surgical Pathology Report

Patient: Snodgrass, Alicia
DOB: 6/9/57
Surgeon: Wilberforce
Date: 12/3/03
Operation: Left radical mastectomy
Date of Surgery: 12/1/03

Gross Description:
Specimen is received in formalin, is moderately well fixed and consists of a 1365 gm white skinned breast with an eccentrically located 0.8 cm diameter nipple and 2.7 cm dark brown areola.

There is a recent partially healed 1.7 cm biopsy incision 2.4 cm from the border of the areola. An axillary fat pad containing numerous lymph nodes is contiguous with one border of the specimen. On serial section at 1.0 cm intervals through the entire specimen a poorly delineated firm white tumor gritty on section is present beneath the recent incision. By visual examination and palpation 17 lymph nodes varying from 1.0-1.3 cm are recovered from the axillary fat pad; on section at least three are grossly partially replaced by tumor. Representative sections are taken from nipple, areola, recent incision, and tumor; all lymph nodes are submitted. Total cassettes with tissue for micro: 28.

Fresh tissue has been submitted prior to fixation for ERA-PRA. (*SCM*)

Microscopic examination:

Sections of nipple, areola, and incision are free of tumor; sections of tumor reveal moderately differentiated adenocarcinoma infiltrating fat; sections of 17 lymph nodes include 5 partially or totally replaced by tumor. (*RLK*)

ERA: positive
PRA: positive.

Pathologic Diagnosis:
Adenocarcinoma gr ii, ductal, with
metastasis to 5 of 17 axillary lymph nodes.

Rufus L. Kirkeness, MD, FACP
Pathologist

A wide variety of diseases may be diagnosed by examination of a tissue specimen, but the diagnosis of cancer is perhaps of greatest concern to most patients. A few definitions will be helpful in understanding terms often used in surgical pathology reports:

adenocarcinoma: a malignant tumor of glandular origin.

adenoma: a benign tumor of glandular origin.

basal cell: a type of skin tumor cell that invades and spreads locally instead of by metastasis to other organs.

benign tumor: a tumor that will not ordinarily spread to other parts of the body or cause death.

blood vessels: the extensive network of arteries, arterioles, veins, and capillaries that transport blood throughout the body.

carcinoma: a malignant tumor made up of cells of epithelial (lining or covering) origin in an organ.

carcinoma-in-situ (CIS): a localized malignant tumor that has not yet spread.

ductal carcinoma: malignant tumor, arising in a glandular organ.

fungating: exuberant tumor growth in a form suggesting a foliated fungus (such as may be seen growing on a tree).

grade: an indication of the aggressiveness— tendency to spread—of tumor cells as seen under the pathologist's microscope; *grade i* is least aggressive, *grade iv* is most aggressive.

invasion: extension of a tumor into adjacent tissues or organs.

-itis: if the diagnosis ends with the suffix "-itis", it means the lesion is inflammatory, not a tumor.

leukemia: a malignancy of white blood cells arsing in the bone marrow or lymph nodes that spreads throughout the body; leukemia may be acute or chronic, and is classified by the type of white blood cell involved, e.g., lymphocytic, monocytic, myelogenous, etc.

local extension: the spread of a tumor into adjacent tissues or organs.

lymphatics: an extensive network of vessels throughout the body that carry a serous fluid, lymph; they do not carry blood, but they connect to lymph nodes, and to blood vessels that can carry tumor cells to other organs.

lymph nodes: small gland-like structures that collect and destroy (when possible) foreign material such as bacteria, fungi, viruses and tumor cells that are traveling in lymphatic vessels, interrupting their spread temporarily or permanently.

malignant tumor: a tumor that can spread locally or distantly in the body; it can cause death if not totally removed or destroyed.

metastasis: (*plural*: **metastases**; *adjective*: **metastatic**) the spread of a tumor to distant tissues or organs; this is a characteristic of most malignant tumors.

—oma: if the diagnosis ends with the suffix "-oma", it means that it is a tumor, either benign or malignant.

polyp: a projecting mass of swollen or tumorous membrane or gland; a polyp may be either benign or malignant.

sarcoma: a malignant tumor of connective tissue origin (e.g., bone, cartilage, or muscle).

sentinel node: a lymph node closest to a malignant tumor, giving evidence of whether or not the tumor has already spread to lymphatics and thus requires further examination and treatment.

squamous cell: a type of skin cell that in a skin tumor may metastasize.

tumor: a mass of tissue that performs no useful function but can interfere with the function of organs; it can be either benign or malignant; most cancers are tumors, but not all tumors are cancerous.

In the United States, the most frequently biopsied organs are bone marrow, breast, cervix, colon, lymph node, prostate, and skin, partly because they are the most accessible. Here are a few examples of frequently diagnosed diseases of these organs:

bone marrow:
  benign: anemia (various types); infections.
  malignant: leukemia; metastatic malignant tumor.

breast:
  benign: ductal adenoma; lipoma.
  malignant: adenocarcinoma; ductal carcinoma.

cervix:
  benign: polyp.
  malignant: squamous cell carcinoma; carcinoma-in-situ ("CIS").

colon:
  benign: colitis; polyp (adenomatous, mucosal, sessile).
  malignant: adenocarcinoma; adenocarcinomatous polyp.

lymph node:
  benign: lymphadenitis
  malignant: lymphoma; leukemia; metastatic malignant tumor.

prostate:
  benign: prostatitis; hypertrophy ("BPH").
  malignant: adenocarcinoma.

skin:

> *benign*: infections; keratosis; senile keratosis; irritated keratosis; solar keratosis (a keratosis may be pre-cancerous).
>
> *malignant*: basal cell carcinoma; squamous cell carcinoma; melanoma.

Any report of a malignant tumor requires discussion with your physician, who may suggest consultation with a general surgeon, a plastic surgeon, a radiologist, an oncologist, or all four.

Bone marrow examination is done for a wide spectrum of reasons related to the presence or absence of infecting organisms, anemias, assessment of the amount of iron stored in the body, blood clotting elements, leukemia, polycythemia (thickened blood), metastatic cancer (a malignant tumor that has spread), and other diseases.

Breast cancer proven by biopsies may be followed by assessment of the hormonal responsiveness of a malignant tumor through use of the estrogen receptor assay (ERA), and the progesterone receptor assay (PRA) (*see Chapter 14, 2.*). These are often helpful in deciding the type of therapy most appropriate for patient management. Still under long-term investigation is the best management of controlling the spread of breast cancer. Whether radical mastectomy, lumpectomy, lumpectomy with sentinel lymph node biopsy, or any of the above combined with hormones, chemotherapeutic agents, radiation, or all of these is best, alone or in various combinations, has still to be resolved by definitive clinical studies. Therefore once the diagnosis is known, all of the options for treatments should be discussed in depth between the patient and her surgeon and an oncologist. Only then can she be an informed participant in deciding which treatment she wants. This ultimately must be the decision of the patient, not her doctor.

Cervical biopsies or Pap smears that are positive for malignancy require immediate attention and follow up. **Cervical carcinoma-in-situ (CIS)** can usually be treated conservatively, without extensive surgery, while **invasive carcinoma of the cervix**, usually of squamous cell variety, can spread upward into the body of the uterus as well as spread into the bladder, rectum, and other parts of the pelvis. These are very serious problems with unpleasant consequences. Early diagnosis of cervical cancer and prevention of spread has been greatly enhanced by the periodic use of the Pap smear (*see Chapter 14, 4.*).

Colon cancer is sometimes detected by using the Occult Blood in the Stool test (*see Chapter 14, 3.*), but increasingly sigmoidoscopy and colonoscopy are used to detect colon cancer in its early stages, usually presenting as a malignant polyp. If a malignant tumor is found, it is removed surgically and its progress, or hopefully the lack of it, can be followed by using the Carcinoembryonic Antigen (CEA) test (*see Chapter 14, 1.*).

Prostatic cancer is very common in older men. Fortunately, in most men it is slow growing and at times behaves in an indolent manner. Many physicians believe that the Prostate Specific Antigen (PSA) test (*see Chapter 14, 5.*) is a useful means for detecting prostatic cancer early enough to allow prevention of its spread to bones and other organs, and also monitoring its progression or response to treatment after it has been diagnosed. Detection of cancer using the PSA test has been very helpful in instituting early treatment. However, great difficulty often arises in the management of a patient with this disease.

Two schemes have been devised to assess the potential behavior of the cancer in relation to the patient's age and in deciding on a choice of therapeutic programs. One of these schemes is *Gleason scoring*. Gleason scoring has been fairly widely accepted as a means of predicting the *prognosis* (how things may turn out) in prostatic cancer. Long-term studies of patients whose prostate cancer has been graded with the

Gleason scoring system, i.e., 1 (good prognosis) to 10 (poor prognosis), have shown a strong correlation of these scores with the long-range life expectancy.

Another system of grading of most cancers, including prostate cancer is *conventional* malignancy grading: the tumor's aggressiveness based on the appearance of the cancer cells and their organization as seen through the microscope. This grading of prostatic cancer by the two methods allows generalizations about a patient's future outlook when the grades of prostatic cancers (malignancy i-iv, and Gleason 1-10) are combined.

If the pathology report states that cancer of the prostate gland is present and conventional malignancy grade is HIGH (grade iii or iv), and Gleason grade is 8-10, one can expect:
a poorly behaving malignant tumor: tumor invasion into nearby tissues or distant spread (metastasis) of the cancer is more likely than not to take place rapidly.
If malignancy grade is INTERMEDIATE (conventional grade ii or iii and Gleason grade 5-7, one can expect:
a moderately-behaving malignant tumor, but tumor behavior is indeterminate—it may or may not spread rapidly.
If malignancy grade is LOW (conventional grade i, and Gleason grade 1-4):
a well-behaving malignant tumor; the spread of prostatic cancer is less likely to be rapid, if at all.

A problem arises when the scores of either (or both) the Gleason and the conventional scores fall into the INTERMEDIATE category: Gleason 5-7, and conventional ii-iii. Tumor behavior is then less predictable than when scores and grades are either in the HIGH or LOW categories.

Management of prostatic cancer (like breast cancer in a woman) is a difficult and perplexing problem for both the patient, his family, and his doctor because of the complications of various approaches to therapy. The prognosis for a patient with prostatic cancer needs to be discussed at length amongst all three parties involved. The often-heard medical aphorism relating to prostatic is worth remembering: "Prostate cancer is *usually* one that a patient dies with, rather than from." Usually, but surely not always. But, as with breast cancer, the patient must make the decision on the treatment course to be undertaken—not his doctor.

Skin cancers—the most common are **basal cell carcinoma, squamous cell carcinoma** and **malignant melanoma**—are usually controllable by early detection and removal by surgical excision. Pre-cancerous keratoses often respond well to cryotherapy (freezing with liquid nitrogen). All three cancers, and especially the first two, are found in sun-exposed parts of the body. Yearly examination of the entire unclothed body (often not done!) is essential for this purpose; this should be part of any periodic health examination, since melanoma may arise in not only sun-exposed skin, but also in obscure areas that can easily be overlooked, such as the sole of the foot, or in genital or anal areas—or even in the retina inside the eye.

Also important and effective is self-examination (remember that early morning health assessment mentioned in Chapter 1?) of the bare body, especially periodically with the help of a partner. The brown or black pigmented skin cancer malignant melanoma is very dangerous—and sometimes deadly—because a small lesion may spread widely before it has been noticed.

Other than biopsy and examination of a lesion under the microscope, there is no reliable laboratory test at present to detect skin cancers early. If spread of *any* type of cancer is suspected by a doctor, examination by X-ray, CAT-scan, MRI, or other means may be necessary before decisions are made concerning therapy. Periodic follow-up appointments with a physician or specialist consultants is strongly advised when cancer is diagnosed.

III

*Interpretations of Medical
Laboratory Test Results*

FOREWORD

This section will help you understand what the medical laboratory test you have had performed actually measures, what the normal range is for the test, the origin of the substance in your body the test is based on, the significance of high test results or low test results, the diagnoses that these test results suggest *(see the "Differential Diagnosis" discussed in Chapter 4 in Part I),* followed by further comments of importance, and what follow-up actions are indicated if your test result is abnormal.

Each test is introduced with a typical symptom, physical complaint or concern a patient might have that the laboratory test addresses, and an illustrative fictitious example of an abnormal test result is shown to indicate if this abnormal test result would require immediate action or perhaps a delayed decision.

The tests for which interpretations are given are those that are most frequently ordered in most clinical laboratories. These include categories of tests for acute and chronic diseases, blood diseases, cancer screens, and heart diseases. Tests appropriate for annual check-ups, for infants, children and adolescents, menopausal women, men with prostrate problems, problems of pregnancy and infertility, sexually transmitted diseases and therapeutic drugs are also included in an easily read and understandable format.

Some test Interpretations may be found listed in more than one of the following chapters. This duplication is intentional. In the interest of reader friendliness, rather than asking the reader to turn back to search for an Interpretation that has already been presented in a previous chapter (e.g. *"see Digoxin, Chapter 16")* the Interpretation has been repeated in the chapter the reader is perusing.

CHAPTER 11

Acute Disease Tests

1. Blood Culture

2. C-Reactive Protein

3. *Giardia lamblia* Parasite

4. Hepatitis Panels

5. Heterophil Antibody

6. HIV1/HIV2 Serology

7. Infectious Mononucleosis ("Mono")

8. Liver Function Panel—Jaundice Screen
Total Bilirubin
Direct (Conjugated) Bilirubin
Prothrombin Time (PT)

9. Liver Function Panel
Alanine Aminotransferase (ALT)
Alkaline Phosphatase
Aspartate Aminotransferase (AST)

Direct (Conjugated) Bilirubin
Gamma Glutamyl Transferase (GGT)
Lactic Dehydrogenase (LDH)
Prothrombin Time (PT)
Total Bilirubin

10. Lyme Disease Serology

11. Ova and Parasites in Stool (O&P)

12. Rapid Plasma Reagin Test (RPR)

13. Stool Culture

14. *Streptococcus* ("Strep") Screen

15. Throat Culture

16. Urethral Culture

17. Urine Culture

18. Vaginal Culture

1. BLOOD CULTURE

TYPICAL WORRY: *I stepped on a nail and I have a swollen foot and a fever. I'm afraid that I might have blood poisoning.*

TEST: Blood culture.

TEST RESULT: *(example)Streptococcus pyogenes.*

URGENCY LEVEL: Action: _√_ Decision: _____

NORMAL RANGE: No growth.

ORIGIN OR SOURCE OF SUBSTANCE TESTED FOR: a microrganism (germ) such as a bacterium or a fungus not normally present in the blood.

DIFFERENTIAL DIAGNOSIS:

If test results show GROWTH of a bacterium or a fungus:

> a blood stream infection ("bacteremia", "blood poisoning") is present; this can be caused by a wide variety of microorganisms; bacteria more common found are *streptococcus, staphylococcus,* and *E. coli*; more common fungi are *candida* and *aspergillus.*

If test results report NO GROWTH:

> a blood stream infection is unlikely.

COMMENT: Blood stream infections (blood poisoning) are serious. *False-negative* culture results are common in preliminary reports. Sometimes it takes several days for a germ to grow and be identified. Viruses will not grow in conventional blood culture media; special procedures are necessary to discover viruses in the blood. Blood culture reports include "Sensitivities", tests that show which antibiotic would work best to kill the disease-causing germ in the blood.

FOLLOW-UP: Call or see your doctor immediately if any microorganism is cultured from your blood, or if you continue to have signs of infection. Your physician will choose any follow-up tests and treatment that may be necessary.

2. C-REACTIVE PROTEIN

TYPICAL WORRY: *I feel lousy. I think I may have an infection somewhere.*

TEST: C-Reactive protein (CRP)

TEST RESULTS: (*example*) 27 mg/ml (SI: 27 mmol/L)

URGENCY LEVEL: Action: __√__ Decision: _____

NORMAL RANGE: < 8 μg/mL (SI: < 8 μmol/L)

ORIGIN OR SOURCE OF SUBSTANCES TESTED FOR: a substance produced in the liver indicating inflammation and/or infection.

DIFFERENTIAL DIAGNOSIS:

If test result is HIGH:

> bacterial infection, viral infection, or inflammation somewhere in the body (higher levels are indicative of *bacterial* infection, lower levels of *viral* infection); rheumatoid arthritis; rheumatic fever; bacteremia (blood poisoning) in infants and toddlers who have high fever.

If test result is LOW:

> neither inflammation nor infection is likely to be present; also indicative of rheumatoid arthritis under good medical control with consequent decreased risk of functional impairment.

COMMENT: The test is very sensitive, but also very non-specific. The test is often overlooked by healthcare providers as a useful screening test when the patient has non-specific complaints of illness or appears to be ill. It may be useful when it is difficult to tell if the patient is one of the worried well, is really ill, or perhaps is malingering. The test may be increasingly used as a a screening test for coronary artery disease; there is evidence in the medical literature that C-Reactive protein elevation may be useful in predicting heart attack and stroke. It is suspected that inflammation of artery walls may be related to the deposition of the fatty substances that clog the coronary (heart) and cerebral (brain) arteries.

CRP has largely replaced the erythrocyte sedimentation rate (ESR), another non-specific screening test for infection or inflammation, although the ESR may be useful in diagnosis of some types of anemia and of some malignant tumors.

FOLLOW-UP: Any evidence of inflammation or infection requires further testing to locate the source with more specific tests; these must be seleceted by a physician based on signs of disease, symptoms, and medical history.

3. *Giardia lamblia* Parasite

TYPICAL WORRY: *I drank brook water while hiking, and now I have diarrhea. Could it be Giardiasis?*

TEST: ELISA testing for *Giardia* antigens in feces.

TEST RESULT: (*example*) Positive.

URGENCY LEVEL: Action: _√_ Decision: _____

NORMAL RANGE: No *Giardia* present; Ova and Parasites: negative.

ORIGIN OR SOURCE OF SUBSTANCE TESTED FOR: a water—borne parasite infesting the gastrointestinal tract, causing foul—smelling diarrhea, flatulence ("farting", "passing gas") and abdominal cramps.

DIFFERENTIAL DIAGNOSIS:

If the test is POSITIVE for *Giardia*:

infestation with the parasite is present.

If test result is NEGATIVE for *Giardia*:

other causes of persistent, foul-smelling and gaseous diarrhea should be sought (*see "Ova and Parasites in Stool Test", and "Stool Culture" in this chapter*).

COMMENT: The test is specific for *Giardia*, a microscopic protozoan flagellate parasite usually entering the gastrointestinal tract by the drinking of contaminated water. Beaver have been suspected, but not proven to be a vector (an organism that spreads a disease) in the spread of the parasite in isolated cases, but other sources have been implicated in epidemics.

FOLLOW-UP: Call your doctor, who may order other tests to discover another cause for your diarrhea if no *Giardia* has been found, or initiate treatment if *Giardia* is present.

4. HEPATITIS PANELS

TYPICAL WORRY: *I have a yellow tint in my eyeballs and I feel lousy. I drink quite a lot. Am I getting hepatitis, or cirrhosis of the liver?*

Hepatitis means inflammation of the liver, and is a disease with serious consequences. There are three tests in the Liver Function Panel—Jaundice Screen, and eight tests in the full Liver Function Panel. The full panel of tests will help detect hepatitis of several types with or without jaundice (yellow jaundice) including hepatitis A and hepatitis B, as well as a particularly chronic form, hepatitis C. Hepatitis A is usually spread by fecal-oral contact (fingers to mouth), especially from fecally contaminated food which is common in countries with impure water supplies (the nice fresh green salad in the dining room of your Nile River cruise vessel may have been washed before it was put before you, but think about the source of the water it may have been washed in!).

Hepatitis B is often spread by unprotected sexual intercourse, and can also be transmitted by exposure to blood infected with the virus. Both hepatitis B and C are frequently transmitted amongst people using illegal street drugs injected with contaminated needles. Hepatitis E is not common in the United States but is prevalent in many other parts of the world.

Diagnosis of specific types of hepatitis may be difficult. A patient's medical history, a careful physical examination, and a panel of liver function tests interpreted by an experienced and skillful physician are often necessary to reach a correct diagnosis.

See in this Chapter: Liver Function Panel—Jaundice Screen, and Liver Function Panel.

5. HETEROPHILE ANTIBODY ("MONO" SCREENING TEST)

TYPICAL WORRY: *Have I got Infectious Mononucleosis ("Mono")?*

TEST RESULT: *(example)* Positive

URGENCY LEVEL: Action: __√__ Decision: _____

NORMAL RANGE: Negative

ORIGIN OR SOURCE OF SUBSTANCE TESTED FOR: antibodies produced within the body's immune system and present in the blood.

DIFFERENTIAL DIAGNOSIS:

If test results are POSITIVE:

> Infectious mononcleosis ("Mono") with or without evidence of liver involvement; some other, less likely diseases: rheumatoid arthritis; infectious hepatitis; lymphoma; leukemia; *false-positive* test results (2%).

If test results are NEGATIVE:

> disease may still be present, giving *false-negative* test results, often because antibodies have not yet been produced by the body's immune system.

COMMENT: Although the prognosis for recovery is good, recovery time may vary from a few weeks to several months. The test for the heterophile antibody may remain positive for many months after symptoms have disappeared, and may be the cause of a *false-positive* serologic test for syphilis (STS). A rapid screening test (Monospot™) is widely used to detect the disease. Liver function tests may indicate liver inflamation when infectious mononuclcosis is present.

FOLLOW-UP: If your test results are Positive, see your physician, who will choose appropriate further tests, if any, that may be necessary.

6. HIV-1/HIV-2 SEROLOGY

TYPICAL WORRY: *I'm afraid I've been exposed to HIV infection.*

TEST: Serologic test for Human Immunodeficiency Viruses (HIV-1 and HIV-2).

TEST RESULT: *(example)* Positive

URGENCY LEVEL: Action: __√__ Decision: _____

NORMAL RANGE: Negative.

ORIGIN OR SOURCE OF SUBSTANCE TESTED FOR: antibodies produced by the body's immune system in response to the HIV infection.

DIFFERENTIAL DIAGNOSIS :

if test results are POSITIVE:

> HIV infection is highly likely, but must be confirmed by a follow-up test (i.e., Western Blot test).

if test results are NEGATIVE:

> infection by HIV is unlikely, but early after exposure the test may be a *false-negative.*

COMMENT: Most, but not necessarily all diseases associated with this test abnormality are HIV-1 or HIV-2 infections, with or without AIDS (Acquired Immunodeficiency Syndrome). The prognosis is better for long time survival if treatment is started early.

Note: If the HIV test is negative after the possibility of exposure is presumed, repeating the test in 2 or 3 weeks is essential, because the antibodies tested for IIIV virus may not yet have been devloped by the body's immune system, although the virus is present and active in the body.

FOLLOW-UP: If your test results are positive, see your physician immediately. Your physician will choose the follow-up tests, if any, that may be necessary. *Advise your sexual partner(s) of your HIV infection if your HIV test is POSITIVE.*

CHAPTER 11

7. INFECTIOUS MONONUCLEOSIS SCREENING TEST

(MONOSPOT™)

TYPICAL WORRY: *I have a bad sore throat and feel lousy. Maybe I've got Infectious Mononucleosis ("I.M.", "Mono").*

(See 5. HETEROPHILE ANTIBODY in this Chapter).

8. LIVER FUNCTION PANEL— JAUNDICE SCREEN

TYPICAL WORRY: *I drink a lot, and I think my eyeballs look a little yellow.*

TESTS: Direct (Conjugated) Bilirubin
Prothrombin Time (PT)
Total Bilirubin

TEST RESULT: (*examples*)
Total Bilirubin : 2.2 mg/dL (SI: 37 mmol/L)
Direct Bilirubin : 1.3 mg/dL (SI: 22 mmol/L)
Prothrombin Time : 18 seconds (SI: same)

URGENCY LEVEL: Action: _√_ Decision: _____

NORMAL RANGE:
Total Bilirubin : 0.3-1.0 mg/dL (SI: 5-17 mmol/L)
Direct Bilirubin: = or < 0.4 mg/dL (SI:= or < 7mmol/L)
Prothrombin Time: 10-13 seconds (SI: same)

ORIGIN OR SOURCE OF SUBSTANCE TESTED FOR: a pigmented substance produced in the liver, stored in the gall bladder, and excreted into the intestinal tract.

DIFFERENTIAL DIAGNOSIS:

If Total Bilirubin is HIGH:

gall bladder disease; liver disease (including cirrhosis and hepatitis); infectious mononucleosis ("Mono"); alcoholism; certain types of anemia (e.g., hemolytic anemia, pernicious anemia).

CHAPTER 11

If Direct Bilirubin is HIGH:

> liver disease, gall bladder disease, bile duct disease (obstruction in the connections between liver, gall bladder, and intestines).

If Prothrombin Time is HIGH:

> liver disease; possible drug effect.

If Total and Direct Bilirubin and Prothrombin Time are LOW:

> no specific significance other than possible drug effect.

COMMENT: The diagnosis of liver disease is often difficult, and requires a physician's evaluation of medical history, signs of disease, symptoms, and laboratory tests. The three tests used as examples in this Liver Panel are frequently used as a starting point in sorting out the underlying liver disease. Prothrombin Time is an especially sensitive test for liver abnormality, although it has low specificity. Bilirubin, both Total and Direct, are the essential tests to begin an evaluation, especially if jaundice is present. Some or all of the other tests listed in the Liver Function Panel (*see in this Chapter, following*) are almost always necessary. If either or both of the Bilirubin test results are abnormal, a physician should be consulted. Jaundice may result from a wide variety of diseases, including alcoholic cirrhosis and gall bladder or bile duct problems.

FOLLOW-UP: If your test results are abnormal for the tests in this Jaundice Screen, or if you note a yellow tinge to the sclera (whites of your eyes) or your skin, see a physician at once. Liver disease is very serious and requires immediate attention.

9. LIVER FUNCTION PANEL

TYPICAL WORRY: *I have a yellow tint in my eyeballs and I drink quite a lot. Am I getting cirrhosis of the liver?*

FREQUENTLY INCLUDED LIVER PANEL TESTS: Alkaline phosphatase (AP), Alanine aminotransferase (ALT), Aspartate aminotransferase (AST), Direct (Conjugated) bilirubin, Ferritin, Gamma Glutamyl Transferase (GGT), Lactic dehydrogenase (LDH), Prothrombin Time (PT), Total bilirubin.

TEST RESULTS: (*examples*)

> AP: HIGH
> ALT: HIGH
> AST: HIGH
> Direct bilirubin: HIGH
> Ferritin: HIGH
> GGT: HIGH
> LDH: HIGH
> PT: PROLONGED
> Total Bilirubin: HIGH.

URGENCY LEVEL: Action: _√_ Decision: _____

NORMAL RANGES: AP: (varies by test method used)

> ALT: (varies by test method used)
> AST: (varies by test method used)
> Direct Bilirubin: = or< 0.4 mg/dL (SI: = or < 7.0 mmol/L)
> Ferritin: *male:* 20-250 ng/mL (SI: 20-250 mg/L)
> *female:* 12-263 ng/mL (SI: 12-263 mg/L)
> GGT: (varies by test method used)
> LDH: < 200 units/L (SI: < 96 IU/L)

PT: 10-13 seconds (SI: same)
Total Bilirubin: 0.3-1.0 mg/dL (SI: 5-17 mmol/L)

ORIGIN OR SOURCE OF SUBSTANCE TESTED FOR:
various enzymes and pigments originating in the liver and circulating in the blood.

DIFFERENTIAL DIAGNOSIS :

If *any* of the above tests are HIGH:

liver disease or liver damage is likely.

If *all* of the test results are LOW or NORMAL:

liver disease is unlikely. Low test results usually are of little or no importance when evaluating most liver function tests.

COMMENT: Interpretation of liver function tests is complicated and often difficult, and requires a knowledgeable and skillful physician experienced in diagnosing and treating liver (hepatic) disease. Gall bladder disease, cirrhosis, viral hepatitis, liver or pancreatic cancer, hemochromatosis, and alcoholism are some of the more common diseases causing abnormal liver function panel tests. (In this fictitious example, there is evidence of serious liver disease, especially since there is clinical evidence of jaundice, e.g., yellow eyeballs). Liver disease is serious, and abnormal liver test results should not be dismissed lightly. Unsuspected or unadmitted alcoholism is a common cause of liver function test abnormalities. The Prothrombin Time is a particularly sensitive test for evidence of liver disease but it is often overlooked as a useful Liver Function Test.

HIGH ferritin levels may also be found in or associated with hyperthyroidism, as well as susceptibility to the acute respiratory distress syndrome (ARDS), a serious lung disease.

FOLLOW UP: A physician should be consulted if any of the Liver Panel tests are more than marginally abnormal. Referral to an internist or an internist sub-specializing in liver disease (hepatologist) may be necessary to establish a specific diagnosis.

10. LYME DISEASE SEROLOGY

TYPICAL WORRY: *My joints ache. I got a tick bite on my leg while hiking several weeks ago, and I wonder if I have Lyme Disease.*

TEST: Blood Serologic Test for *Borrelia burgdorfi.*

TEST RESULTS: (*example*) Positive

URGENCY LEVEL: Action: __√__ Decision: _____

NORMAL RANGE: Negative

ORIGIN OR SOURCE OF SUBSTANCE TESTED FOR: antibodies produced by the body's immune system to the organism *Borrelia burgdorfi* (anti-Bb) after a deer tick (*Ixodes dammini*) bite.

DIFFERENTIAL DIAGNOSIS:

If test results are POSITIVE:

> an immune response to *Borrelia burgdorfi* is present; recent or past exposure to the organism causing Lyme disease.

If test results are NEGATIVE,

> probably (but not definitely) Lyme Disease is not present.

COMMENT: This test is difficult to interpret without clinical evidence of Lyme Disease, some symptoms of which are subtle. Also, a history of recent exposure and recollection of a tick bite in a part of the country where the deer tick is prevalent is helpful. The deer tick is quite small, unlike the more common and larger tick, *Dermacenter andersoni*, which *does not* transmit *Borrelia* or cause Lyme Disease.

FOLLOW-UP: If the test is POSITIVE, see your doctor, who may order that the test be repeated, or prescribe treatment immediately.

11. OVA AND PARASITES IN STOOL

TYPICAL WORRY: *I've had persistent diarrhea since my trip to Africa.*

TEST: Ova and Parasites in Stool

TEST RESULTS: (*example*) Positive for *E. histolytica*

URGENCY LEVEL: Action: __√__ Decision: ____

NORMAL RANGE: Negative for Ova and Parasites

ORIGIN OR SOURCE OF SUBSTANCES TESTED FOR: one or more parasites or ameba infesting the gastrointestinal tract, usually causing diarrhea.

DIFFERENTIAL DIAGNOSIS:

If test result is POSITIVE:

> Infestation by one or more of the frequently encountered organisms in the stool causing diarrhea, including parasites such as *Giardia lamblia; Cryptosporidium* (frequently found in AIDS patients) *E. histolytica* (causes amebic dysentery, a serious infestation); *Blastocystis hominis* (may not cause significant symptoms); *Isospora belli; Strongyloides stercoralis; Taenia* (tapeworm).

If test result is NEGATIVE or NONE FOUND:

> No parasitic organisms present, but examination of a single stool specimen only may give a *false-negative* test result.

COMMENT: If test result is NEGATIVE, other causes of diarrhea should be sought (*see STOOL CULTURE in this Chapter*); bacterial and viral organisms will not be detected in the OVA AND PARASITES IN STOOL test).

FOLLOW-UP: Call your doctor, who may order that the OVA AND PARASITES IN STOOL test be performed on at least three stools specimens to reduce the likelihood of *false-negative* test results. Other tests to discover the cause of the diarrhea may be ordered. Diarrhea can occur for a wide variety of reasons not associated with parasitic infestation or bacterial or viral infection.

12. RAPID PLASMA REAGIN (RPR) TEST

TYPICAL WORRY: *I have been sexually active and I suspect my last partner may have a venereal disease.*

TEST: Rapid Plasma Reagin (RPR) Test for Syphilis.

RESULTS: (*example*) Positive.

URGENCY LEVEL: Action: __√__ Decision: _____

NORMAL RANGE: Negative

ORIGIN OR SOURCE OF SUBSTANCE TESTED FOR: a substance produced by the body in response to syphilis (and other infections).

DIFFERENTIAL DIAGNOSIS:

If the report is POSITIVE:

> syphilis; many *false-positive* reactions, including: autoimmune diseases (*e.g.*, rheumatoid arthritis; systemic lupus erythematosus); pregnancy; old age; viral infection (*e.g.*, infectious mononucleosis, hepatitis); drug addiction; parasitic diseases (*e.g.*, malaria).

If the report is NEGATIVE:

> no disease; (may be *false-negative* in late stage of syphilis).

COMMENT: Syphilis in the acute stage is revealed as a *chancre*, an ulcerative lesion on the genitalia. This acute stage progresses to a secondary stage manifested by a skin rash, followed, often months or years later, by the third stage, sometimes manifested as a brain tumor (gumma), heart valve lesion, or an aortic aneurysm. The RPR test becomes positive at indeterminate time, and therefore is listed here as an acute disease test. The test has very low specificity, but is more sensitive than a formerly-used screening test, the Venereal Disease Research Laboratory (VDRL) test. Many drugs and a wide variety of infections can cause a *false-positive* RPR test. A POSITIVE test for syphilis is a panic value in pregnancy.

FOLLOW UP: A POSITIVE test result requires immediate evaluation by a physician and a follow-up test, usually FTA-ABS. Syphilis is a treatable disease, especially in its early stages. A NEGATIVE test result does not necessarily mean that disease is not present; *false-negatives* can occur, or the disease may be in an early stage, before reagin has been produced by the body.

13. STOOL CULTURE

TYPICAL WORRY: *I've had severe, persistent bloody diarrhea and fever following my trip to Asia. I'm sure I picked up a bad bug.*

TEST: Stool culture for bacteria

TEST RESULTS: (*example*) Culture: Positive for *Campylobacter* and *Salmonella*

URGENCY LEVEL: Action: __√__ Decision: _____

NORMAL RANGE: Normal flora, No growth, or Negative.

ORIGIN OR SOURCE OF SUBSTANCES TESTED FOR: one or more bacteria not ordinarily present tin the gastrointestinal tract, causing an infection.

DIFFERENTIAL DIAGNOSIS:
If the bacterial culture is POSITIVE:

> dysentery, bacterial origin; colitis.

If the bacterial culture is NEGATIVE:

> inflammatory bowel disease; irritable bowel syndrome; other causes of symptoms such as parasitic infestation.

COMMENT: Gastroenteritis with vomiting is usually due to vial infection or caused by the bacteria *Staphylococcus* or *Bacillus cereus* as a result of food poisoning, whereas watery, large volume stools are indicative of enteritis (small bowel infection) that may be caused by the bacterium *Vibrio cholerae* or some strains of *E. coli.* Colitis (inflammation of the large bowel) is usually due to an ameba such as *E. histolytica,* or a parasite. Neither parasites nor ameba will grow in a culture of the stool for bacteria, but will be detected by the OVA AND PARASITES IN STOOL test for bacteria such as *Shigella, Salmonella* or *Campylobacter* (*see 11. Ova and Parasites in Stool test in this Chapter*). However, colitis or enteritis may be due to inflammatory or irritable bowel disease, or ulcerative colitis rather than any of the infectious agents mentioned above.

FOLLOW-UP: Call your doctor, who may order other tests to make a specific diagnosis. Effective treatment requires identification of the microorganism(s) (germs) causing the symptoms.

14. *STREPTOCOCCUS* ("STREP ") SCREEN

TYPICAL WORRY: *My baby has a really bad sore throat. Maybe she has a strep throat.*

TEST: Strep Screen and Throat Culture Screen for *Streptococcus* Group A hemolytic (*Streptococcus pyogenes*).

TEST RESULT: (*example*) Screen: Positive for *Streptococcus pyogenes*.

URGENCY LEVEL: Action: __√__ Decision:

NORMAL RANGE: Negative; Culture: Normal flora

ORIGIN OR SOURCE OF SUBSTANCES TESTED FOR: a bacterium not ordinarily present in the throat that can cause a serious infection.

DIFFERENTIAL DIAGNOSIS:

If the screening test or culture is POSITIVE:

> *Streptococcus pyogenes* is present and probably is causing the infection.

If the screening test or culture is NEGATIVE:

> in the presence of a sore throat, possible presence of any of a variety of viral or fungal organisms that can cause a sore throat.

COMMENT: Strep screens are ordinarily only useful for detecting *Streptococcus pyogenes;* a THROAT CULTURE (*see next in this Chapter*) may detect many other bacteria that inhabit the throat and mouth, most of which do not cause infection. A NEGATIVE screen in a patient with a sore throat should be followed up by culture of the throat for other bacteria, and/or a screening test for Infectious Mononucleosis ("Mono") (*see in this Chapter*). Viruses and some bacteria require special culture methods for detection.

FOLLOW-UP: Call or see your doctor, who may either start antibiotic treatment if either the STREP SCREEN or THROAT CULTURE is POSITIVE, or order other tests to detect viruses or fungi that may be causing the sore throat. Fungus infection of the mouth and throat may indicate testing for SEXUALLY TRANSMITTED DISEASE (STD) in patients known or suspected to be at risk for these diseases (*see tests 6, 12, 16 and 18, this Chapter*).

15. THROAT CULTURE

TYPICAL WORRY: *I have a wicked sore throat; I'm hoarse and I'm having trouble swallowing but I don't have a cough.*

TEST: Throat Culture

TEST RESULT: (*example*) *Staphylococcus aureus*, coagulase positive.

URGENCY LEVEL: Action: __√__ Decision: _____

NORMAL RANGE: "No growth", "Normal flora" "Usual throat flora", "No pathogenic organisms", or "Negative for bacteria and fungi".

ORIGIN OR SOURCE OF SUBSTANCES TESTED FOR: bacteria ("germs") or fungi not ordinarily present in the throat that can cause an infection.

DIFFERENTIAL DIAGNOSIS:

If the screening test or culture is POSITIVE:

> pathogenic (disease-causing) bacteria or fungus present.

If the screening test or culture is NEGATIVE:

> possible presence of viral organisms that could cause a sore throat, but would not be discovered in a culture for bacteria.

COMMENT: A throat culture many detect many microorganisms that inhabit the mouth and throat, many of which do not cause infection. The number of diseases manifested by the symptom of a sore throat is large and includes peritonsillar abscess, viral pharyngitis (inflammation of the throat), gingivitis (inflammation of the gums), infectious mononucleosis ("I.M.", "Mono"; *see test 5 this Chapter*), tonsillitis, roseola (febrile disease accompanied by a rash, common in children), sinusitis, "thrush" (infection by the fungus *Candida albicans*), strep throat caused by *Streptococcus pyogenes* ("Strep") (*see test14 in this Chapter*)—to name a few of those that are more common.

If the sore throat is accompanied by a cough, other diseases such as the common cold, influenza (flu), laryngitis, and measles (usually a childhood disease) may be the underlying cause of the symptoms.

A NEGATIVE culture in a patient with a persistent sore throat that doesn't respond to antibiotics should be followed up by culture of the throat for unusual microorganisms and/or the screening test for infectious mononucleosis. Viruses, some bacteria and other microorganisms require special tests for their detection.

FOLLOW-UP: Call or see your doctor, who may either start antibiotic treatment if either the STREP SCREEN or THROAT CULTURE is POSITIVE for a disease-causing organism, or order other tests to detect viruses or fungi that may be causing the sore throat. Fungus infection of the mouth and throat may indicate testing for SEXUALLY TRANSMITTED DISEASE (STD) in patients known or suspected to be at risk for these diseases (*see tests 6, 12, 16 and 18, this Chapter*).

16. URETHRAL CULTURE

TYPICAL WORRY: *I've had recent unprotected sex with a girl who I thought was clean—but now I have a drip from my penis and it stings when I piss.*

TEST: Urethral bacterial culture (or DNA Detection Test on the penile discharge fluid).

TEST RESULT: (*example*) Positive for *Neisseria gonorrheae*

URGENCY LEVEL: Action: __√__ Decision: _____

NORMAL RANGE: Negative, or No growth.

ORIGIN OR SOURCE OF SUBSTANCES TESTED FOR: a bacterium not ordinarily present in the urethra, bladder, or genital organs.

DIFFERENTIAL DIAGNOSIS:

If the bacterial culture is POSITIVE for *Neisseria gonorrheae*:

> definitive evidence of gonorrhea ("the clap"); if the test used was *Neisseria gonorrhea* DNA Detection Test and the test result was positive, infection is most likely present.

If the bacterial culture is NEGATIVE for *Neisseria gonorrheae*,

> infection may still be present because of the difficulty in culturing this bacterium, possibly resulting in a false-negative report; if the test used was *Neisseria gonorrhea* DNA Detection Test and the test result was negative, infection is unlikely.

COMMENT: A urethral culture is taken to detect infection of the male and female sex organs, and it is often referred to as a "Genital Culture". When *Neisseria gonorrheae* infection is present, *Chlamydia trachomatis* may also be present; even if *Neisseria* is not found, *Chlamydia* infection may still be present, often without symptoms. If either of these organisms infects a female and is unsuspected, undetected, and untreated, it may cause salpingitis (inflammation of the fallopian tubes), ectopic (tubal) pregnancy, or infertility, or all three.

FOLLOW-UP: Call or see your doctor, who will prescribe treatment and may order additional tests to make sure other sexually transmitted diseases (STD) such as HIV and syphilis are not also present.

17. URINE CULTURE

TYPICAL WORRY: *I have burning when I urinate, and I have to go all the time; I've had this before, and I'm pretty sure I've got cystitis again.*

TEST: Culture of urine for bacteria ("Random Clean Catch" Culture)

TEST RESULT: (*example*) Positive for *E.coli.*

URGENCY LEVEL: Action: __√__ Decision: _____

NORMAL RANGE: less than (<) 1000 CFU (culture forming units), or Negative.

ORIGIN OR SOURCE OF SUBSTANCES TESTED FOR: microorganisms ("germs") present in the urinary tract (bladder, urethra, ureters, kidneys).

DIFFERENTIAL DIAGNOSIS:

If the bacterial culture is POSITIVE:

> bacteria: urinary tract infection (UTI);
> fungus: *Candida albicans (C. albicans)*, a common contaminant of urine specimens, may give a false positive test result, but *C. albicans* and other fungi may also be causative of disease.

If the culture is NEGATIVE:

> bacterial or fungal infection is unlikely.

COMMENT: *E.coli* is the most common bacterium associated with cystitis in females. Other cause of UTI symptoms may be viral infection, bladder or kidney stones, or prolapse ("falling down") of the uterus. The urine specimen is best collected in the morning, and at the laboratory where the test is to be done so that an uncontaminated fresh specimen will be obtained. Some laboratories use a technique of staining a small amount of urine and examining it under the microscope for a quick evaluation of whether or not bacteria, fungi, or parasites are present. A culture of the urine will identify specific microorganisms, allowing a physician to choose the proper medication for treatment.

UTI can be serious, and is often the source of blood stream infection, especially in the elderly. Therefore any UTI deserves immediate medical attention. UTIs are a common cause of serious complications and sometimes death following hip fracture surgery in the elderly.

FOLLOW-UP: Call or see your doctor, who will prescribe treatment and may order additional tests to make a specific diagnosis of any possible disease underlying the symptoms such as diabetes, kidney infection, stones in the urinary tract, or other problem.

18. VAGINAL CULTURE

TYPICAL WORRY: *I have a heavy and smelly vaginal discharge; I have had herpes infection in the past, and I'm pregnant.*

TEST: Vaginal bacterial/fungal culture of discharge

TEST RESULT: (*example*) Culture: *Candida albicans*

URGENCY LEVEL: Action: __√__ Decision: _____

NORMAL RANGE: "Normal flora"; "No growth"; "Negative".

ORIGIN OR SOURCE OF SUBSTANCE TESTED FOR: microorganisms (bacteria, fungus, parasite) not ordinarily present in the vagina and causing infection

DIFFERENTIAL DIAGNOSIS:

If the culture result is POSITIVE:

> for: *Candida albicans,* yeast vaginitis ("thrush", or "the whites"), the most common cause of discharge due to vaginal infection;
> for: *Chlamydia trachomatis; Neisseria gonorrhea; Streptococcus, Group B;* or *Ureaplasma urealyticum*: a bacterial infection by one or more of these bacteria.

If the culture result is NEGATIVE:

> an infecting agent may still be present e.g., viruses such as *Herpes simplex* (*HSV1 and HSV2*) or *Cytomegalus* (*CMV*), or parasites such as *Trichomonas*—which will not be detected by the standard bacterial and fungal

culture techniques but can be detected by "wet mount prep" or Pap smear.

COMMENT: A "wet mount prep" is a quick, inexpensive screening test often used in laboratories for detecting *Trichomonas* (a parasite) and *Candida* albicans (a fungus). Strand Displacement Amplification (SDA) testing and urine cultures may be used in place of the conventional culture of vaginal secretions. Testing for microorganisms can often be less expensive when performed or ordered at a Sexually Transmitted Disease (STD) Clinic.

Teen-agers are often afraid to tell their parents or go to a doctor when they have symptoms or worries about STD or pregnancy. Walk-in Family Planning Clinics (FPC) staffed by friendly and understanding female nurses in a non-intimidating setting are often a solution to this vexing personal, social, and public health problem.

FOLLOW UP: Many infections that are known to be sexually transmitted diseases *must* be reported to local or state health departments. Treatment for these diseases requires medical expertise, since some untreated STDs may lead to problems of a chronic nature, including infertility.

Call your doctor, who may order other tests to make a specific diagnosis. Newer, highly sensitive tests for many microorganisms are now available that use techniques of molecular biology such as *DNA probes.* These tests are characteristically more expensive than standard culture tests, but when suspicion of infection is high and usual culture test results are negative, they may be worth the greater expense, given the possible serious complications mentioned above.

CHAPTER 12

Annual Check-Up Tests

1. Cholesterol

2. Complete Blood Count (CBC)

3. Lead

4. Occult Blood in Stool (Hemoccult™)

5. Papanicalou Smear

6. Prostate Specific Antigen (PSA)

7. Random Blood Sugar

8. Thyroid Stimulating Hormone (TSH)

9. Urinalysis with Microscopic Examination
(UA with Micro)

1. CHOLESTEROL

TYPICAL WORRY: *I wonder if my cholesterol is high. I'm concerned because both my father and my brother have had heart attacks.*

TEST: Blood cholesterol and cholesterol fractions (high density lipoproein cholesterol, HDLC, and low density lipoprotein cholesterol, LDLC)

TEST RESULTS: (*example is for a 38 year old male*)
Total cholesterol (TC): 225mg/dL (SI: 5.8 mmol/L)
Cholesterol fractions:

High density lipoprotein cholesterol (HDLC, "good" cholesterol): 23 mg/dL (SI: 0.6 mmol/L)
Low density lipoprotein cholesterol (LDLC, "bad" cholesterol): 133 mg/dL (SI: 3.4 mmol/L)
TC to HDLC ratio: 9.78
LDLC to HDLC ratio: 5.78

URGENCY LEVEL: Action: _√_ Decision: _____

AGE-RELATED NORMAL RANGES:

Table 7
**Age-related Approximate Normal Ranges and Ratios
for Cholesterol and Cholesterol Fractions**

SI values in ( )

Age:	0-19	20-29	30-39	>39
TC mg/dL.:	155 (4.0)	175 (4.5)	195 (5.1)	210 (5.4)
HDLC mg/dL:	50 (1.3)	45 (1.2)	45 (1.2)	50 (1.3)
LDLC mg/dL:	95 (2.5)	110 (3.2)	130 (3.4)	145 (3.9)

TC:HDLC:	*male: 3.4 - 9.5;*	*female: 3.3 - 6.9*
LDHC:HDLC:	*male: 2.3 - 4.9;*	*female: 2.3 - 4.1*

ORIGIN OR SOURCE OF SUBSTANCES TESTED FOR:
substances produced by cells in the body; blood levels
can be influenced by genetics, diet, exercise, chronic
alcohol ingestion, hormones, or medications.

DIFFERENTIAL DIAGNOSIS:

If the test results are HIGH:

primary hyperlipoproteinemia (an inherited
predisposition); secondary hyperlipoproteinemia due to kidney disease;
hypothyroidism; diabetes; high fat diet; obesity; lack
of exercise; use of drugs such as steroids, beta
blockers, thiazides.

If the test results are very LOW:

severe liver disease; malabsorption of dietary nutrients;
malnutrition; hyperthryroidism; very old age.

COMMENT: In a nutshell, your total cholesterol should be
below 200, your LDLC("LDL", "bad cholesterol")
should be below 129, the lower the better, and your
HDLC("HDL", "good cholesterol") should be above
50, the higher the better. The LDL Cto HDLC ratios
should be about 2 to 1 or lower, but all of the above
are age-dependent, as can be seen in the *Age—Related
Normal Ranges* in *Table 7.*
All persons under age 20 should have their Total Cholesterol
tested at least once as a screening test to detect a possible
genetic predisposition to coronary artery disease, and
thereafter tested every five years. Those found to have
abnormally high cholesterol should have a Cardiac Risk
Analysis (*see Chapter 16, Heart Disease Tests*) performed

to find abnormalities early enough so that protective measures can be taken to prevent the development of coronary artery or other vascular disease. Table 8 indicates "cardiac risk"related to total cholesterol and high density lipoprotein cholesterol.

Table 8

**Cardiac Risk Based on TC:HDLC Ratio
(Total Cholesterol divided
by High Density Lipoprotein Cholesterol)**

Risk Level	Male	Female
½ average	3.4-4.9	3.3-4.3
average	5.0-9.5	4.4-6.9
2 X average	9.6-23.3	7.0-10.9
3 X average	> 23.3	> 10.9

Average values for Americans are higher than average values for many other geographically or ethnically distinct groups of people worldwide. American average values would be considered abnormally high to physicians in many other parts of the world.

Only one of the cholesterol fraction test results may be abnormal while others are within normal range. Concentrating on improving *any* abnormal values so that all test results fall within normal range is a reasonable goal.

It is now clear that "statins", prescription drugs that lower cholesterol, are very helpful in lowering high cholesterol, especially when combined with appropriate life style behavior.

Antihypertensive medication (*except calcium channel blockers*) may have influence on test results. If you are on such drugs, check with your doctor about the significance of your medications regarding your cholesterol.

FOLLOW-UP: Call or see your doctor for advice if your test results are outside normal ranges. Be sure to discuss any test abnormalities and their possible relationship to your medications.

2. COMPLETE BLOOD COUNT (CBC)

TYPICAL WORRY: *My face is very red and my skin is pinker than it used to be.*

TEST: Complete Blood Count. This will include at least five tests:

> hemoglobin (Hb);
> hematocrit (percentage of the blood composed of
>   red blood cells) (Hct);
> white blood cell (leukocyte) count (WBC);
> red blood cell (erythrocyte) count (RBC);
> platelet (thrombocyte) count (Plts).

Cell indices (MCV, MCH, MCHC, RDW) may also be included; these will be meaningful and important to your doctor if the Hb, Hct, or RBC (or all three) are abnormal.

A Blood Smear Review with WBC differential (the percentage of various types of leukocytes in the blood) is often also included.

TEST RESULTS: (*example*)
> Hb: 17.3 gm/L (SI: 0.93 gm/L)
> Hct: 53%
> RBC: 6,765,000 /cu mm (SI: 6,765,000 x10^{12}/L)
> WBC: 3,750 /cu mm (SI: 3.75x10^9 /L)
> Plt: 112,000/cu mm (SI: 112,000 x10^9/L)
> Smear Review:
> WBC differential: WNL;
> RBC: normocytic and normochromic; Plts: decreased.

URGENCY LEVEL: Action: _√_ Decision: _____

NORMAL RANGES:

Hb: (*female*) 12.7-14.7 gm/dL (SI: 127-147 g/L)
(*male*) 14.7-16. 7 gm/dL (SI: 147-167 g/L)
Hct: (*adult female*) 38-44 %
(*adult male*) 43-49%
RBC: (*female*) 3.5-5.0 106/cu mm (SI: 3.5-5.0 x 10^{12}/L)
(*male*) 4.3-5.9 106/cu mm (SI: 4.3-5.9 x 10^{12}/L)
WBC: 3,200-9,800 /cu mm (SI: 3.2-9.8 x 10^{9}/L)
Plts: 150,000-450,000/cu mm (SI: 150-450 x 10^{9}/L)
Smear Review: "WNL"; "Normal"; "Unremarkable"

ORIGIN OR SOURCE OF SUBSTANCE TESTED FOR: blood cells produced in the body's hematopoietic (blood-producing) system, the bone marrow, spleen, thymus gland and lymph nodes.

DIFFERENTIAL DIAGNOSIS:

If test results are HIGH:

a. Hb, Hct and/or RBCs: polycythemia (too many red blood cells) may be present as a result of dehydration, or an overproduction of red blood cells by the bone marrow;

b. WBCs: may indicate an infection or inflammatory process, bone marrow disease, or leukemia (uncontrolled production of white blood cells by the hematopoietic organs);

c. Plts: thrombocythemia (over-production of thrombocytes in the bone marrow) with consequent thrombosis (stoppage of blood flow by a clot in a blood vessel), a common cause of stroke and heart attack, or artery blockage elsewhere in the body with serious consequences.

If test results are LOW:

for Hb, Hct, or RBC: anemia is present because of:

    a. blood loss,

    b. a failure of the bone marrow to produce enough, or normal, red blood cells,

    c. an abnormal destruction of red blood cells in the body, or

    d. a genetic abnormality (*see Chapter 13, Anemia, Red Blood Cell Abnormalities and Polycythemia*);

for WBCs: may indicate a viral infection or a bone marrow disorder;

for Plts: thrombocytopenia (under-production or loss of thrombocytes); may suggest a blood clotting disorder.

COMMENT: The WBC and Plt count in the CBC are unrelated to anemia in most instances. If the CBC does report these parts of the test to be abnormal as well as the RBC portions, there may be a serious bone marrow disorder. Not all laboratories include a Smear Review or Differential WBC, (the examination of a stained thin layer of blood under the microscope), or is automatically performed by a special laboratory instrument. The differential report includes the percentage of the different types of white blood cells in the blood sample: polymorphonuclear leukocytes (polys), lymphocytes (lymphs), monocytes (monos), eosinophils (eos), and basophils (basos) as well as thrombocytes (platelets).

    Some laboratories may only perform the Smear Review on specific order by the doctor. Any significant abnormality in the Smear Review should be interpreted by a physician. The Smear Review is often omitted from the CBC because it is said to be "not cost-effective" (i.e., not enough "bang-for-the-buck" from an HMO's or insurance company's point of view) ; nevertheless, the blood smear may provide important information helpful in diagnosis (e.g., viral infections, parasite infestation, allergies, infectious mononucleosis, etc.).

Proper treatment of hematological diseases depends on finding the exact cause of the disease. For instance, not all anemias respond to iron medication, and only rarely (when pernicious anemia is diagnosed) are injections of vitamin B_{12} helpful; each of the many types of anemia requires treatment specific for the type of anemia diagnosed. (*See in Chapter 13, "Anemias, Red Blood Cell Abnormalities and Polycythemia" a broader discussion of various hematologic disorders revealed by abnormal test results in the CBC*).

FOLLOW-UP: See your doctor for evaluation of any abnormal test result in the CBC. He or she may order that the test be repeated, or initiate an investigation to find the specific cause for the abnormality. This may involve taking a variety of tests.

3. LEAD

TYPICAL WORRY: *I live in an old house and my baby eats everything.*

TEST: Lead (test done on serum from blood)

TEST RESULT: (*example*) 37 mg/dL (SI: 1.8 mmol/L)

URGENCY LEVEL: Action: __√__ Decision: _____

NORMAL RANGE: less than (<) 10 mg/dL

ORIGIN OR SOURCE OF SUBSTANCE TESTED FOR: a chemical element found everywhere in industrial society: soil, air, dust, paint, drinking water, food, exhaust fumes, "moonshine", automobile batteries, many folk remedies.

DIFFERENTIAL DIAGNOSIS:

If blood Lead is HIGH:

lead poisoning (plumbism); mental retardation, and "failure to thrive" in infants and children.

If blood Lead is LOW:

of no significance.

COMMENT: Lead is often an unappreciated occupational and environmental hazard causing varying symptoms; toxicity is rarely suspected (and thus infrequently tested for except in high-risk industries); *it is also an often unsuspected cause of retardation or "failure to thrive" in infants and children.* Minute old paint dust or chips may each contain thousands of micrograms (mg) of lead, and often are the source of lead toxicity. Industrial atmospheric pollutants containing lead are an increasing hazard to health in many localities in the U.S. and other industrialized countries.

FOLLOW-UP: Elevated blood levels require searching for the source of the pollutant, as well as obtaining medical care immediately, especially when elevations are found in infants and children. Current advice is that infants and children should be checked for evidence of elevated blood (serum) lead levels *at least once a year* up to at least age five years to prevent or arrest serious irreversible consequences of lead poisoning, such as mental retardation.

4. OCCULT BLOOD IN THE STOOL

TYPICAL WORRY: *I know cancer of the colon is common and my father died from it. I've never had a test to see if I might be getting it too.*

TEST: Guaic test for Occult (hidden) Blood

TEST RESULT: (*example*) Positive for occult blood.

URGENCY LEVEL: Action: __√__ Decision: _____

NORMAL RANGE: Negative for occult blood.

ORIGIN OR SOURCE OF SUBSTANCES TESTED FOR: Blood leaking into the esophagus or intestinal tract in an amount too small to be noticed in the stool (feces, shit).

DIFFERENTIAL DIAGNOSIS:

If the screening test or culture is POSITIVE:

> bleeding into the esophago-gastrointestinal tract (i.e., from the back of the mouth to the anus; it includes the esophagus, the stomach, the small intestine, the large intestine, rectum and anus).

If the screening test or culture is NEGATIVE:

> no bleeding into the esophago-gastrointestinal tract.

COMMENT: The test has *low specificity* and *low sensitivity (for what these terms mean, see Part I, Chapter 8)*, so there are often *false-positives* and *false-negatives*. However, it is the simplest and least expensive screening test for sources of bleeding somewhere in the entire gastrointestinal tract. The bleeding could come from ulcers, polyps, cancer, or varicose veins at the gastroesophageal junction (where the sophagus connects with the stomach) that have ruptured.

Test kits are available (e.g., Hemoccult™) for detecting small amounts of blood, and most frequently used as a screening test for colon cancer; kit instructions have to be followed carefully to avoid *false-positive* test results. Death from colon cancer is currently second only to lung cancer in the United States. Early detection can lead to proper treatment and often to complete cure by surgical removal of a cancer or a pre-cancerous polyp.

FOLLOW-UP: If blood is found in the stool, notify your doctor at once. Colonoscopy or other procedures often are necessary as an immediate first step in follow-up of a report of blood in the stool in order to rule out cancer of the colon or other lesions in the gastrointestinal tract.

5. PAPANICALOU CYTOLOGIC TEST ("PAP SMEAR")

TYPICAL WORRY: *I haven't had a Pap Smear for many years, and I know I should, there's so much cancer around.*

TEST: Papanicalou Cytologic Test

TEST RESULTS: (*example*) Atypical squamous cells of undetermined significance ("ASCUS")

URGENCY LEVEL: Action: __√__ Decision: _____

NORMAL RANGE: Normal smear

ORIGIN OR SOURCE OF SUBSTANCES TESTED FOR: cells lining the vagina, cervix and inside of the uterus, mixed with secretions.

DIFFERENTIAL DIAGNOSIS:

If the report is POSITIVE:

> for *squamous cell carcinoma*: cancer of cervix or vagina;
> for *adenocarcinoma*: cancer of the cells lining the inside of the uterus or cervix;
> for *carcinoma-in-situ (CIS)*: localized squamous cell cancer of the cervix or vagina.

If the report is ASCUS or *low-grade squamous intraepithelial lesion (LSIL)*:

> the cause is usually indeterminate, but may result from inflammation, having given birth recently, recent sexual intercourse, or menopause.

If the report is NEGATIVE:

no evidence of cancer in this one smear.

COMMENT: A history of having one or more episodes of sexually transmitted disease (STD), human papilloma virus infection, or having begun sexual intercourse early in adolescence all increase the susceptibility of the female to the development of cervical cancer.

FOLLOW-UP: Studies have shown that it may take up to 7 years for cancer to develop after a Pap report of ASCUS or LSIL, although some carcinomas develop much more rapidly. Your doctor may recommend colposcopy (an examination with an instrument that allows close visual inspection of the surface of the vagina and cervix) and biopsy of suspicious lesions as a next step in evaluation (*see Chapter10, "Your Surgical Pathology Biopsy Report"*).

An example of one strategy for follow-up, related to the patient's age and menstrual status:

Post-menopausal: your doctor may prescribe estrogen cream and a repeat of the Pap test (smear) in several months. and then schedule you for yearly Pap tests. Some doctors will recommend proceeding with immediate biopsy.

Pre-menopausal and *post-menopausal* women on hormone replacement therapy (HRT): your doctor may order a repeat of the Pap smear every 4 to 6 months; if three consecutive smears are normal, your doctor might order that Pap smears be done yearly thereafter—although this is a decison to be made by you only after obtaining your doctor's advice.

A POSITIVE or POSITIVE FOR MALIGNANCY report requires *immediate* action to establish a diagnosis by biopsy, followed by appropriate treatment.

6. PROSTATE SPECIFIC ANTIGEN (PSA)

TYPICAL WORRY: *My father and my brother have prostate cancer and so I'm really worried about prostate gland cancer.*

TEST: Prostate Specific Antigen (PSA).

TEST RESULT: (*example*) *22.0* ng/mL

URGENCY LEVEL: Action: __√__ Decision: _____

NORMAL RANGE: Thresholds for possible further investigation:

Total PSA:

> Age: 40's: 2.5 ng/mL
> 50's: 3.5 ng/mL
> 60's: 4.0 ng/mL
> 70+: less than (<) 4.5 ng/mL.

ORIGIN OR SOURCE OF SUBSTANCE TESTED FOR: a protein, including both "bound", and "unbound-to-protein" ("free PSA") portions, produced only by cells in the prostate gland.

DIFFERENTIAL DIAGNOSIS:

If test results are HIGH:

> cancer of the prostate gland;
> benign prostatic hypertrophy (BPH);
> inflammation of the prostate gland (prostatitis).

If test results are LOW:

> prostate cancer is unlikely (a small or localized
>   cancer cannot be absolutely ruled out);
> post-prostatectomy, or after any other treatment (e.g.,
>   radiation) for prostate cancer that has partially
>   or completely destroyed the prostate gland;
> falsely low, due to drug therapy for benign (non-
>   cancerous) enlargement of the prostate gland
>   (BPH); (see Comment following).

COMMENT: Some studies have shown that seventy percent of men between the ages of 50 and 70 years have a PSA below 2.0 ng/mL. Low test results may be due to medication (e.g., Proscar™; Avodart™) for prostate enlargement; be sure your doctor is informed if you are taking these drugs.

The rate of change ("velocity") of the PSA over time is significant; an increase of 0.8 ng/mL/year over three years is evidence that cancer may be present even if the test results remain within the normal range. Although PSA testing is useful, there is an appreciable number of *false-negative* test results (i.e., when the test results fall between the normal range (2.6-4.5 ng/mL) but undetected cancer is present); thus testing annually or every two years is reasonable.

Any rise of the PSA from post-treatment low levels may indicate persistence or recurrence of the cancer.

If the PSA testing is done soon after a digital rectal examination ("DRE") of the prostate gland, there may be further elevation of the test results, but usually only if the test result is markedly elevated to begin with (i.e., >20 ng/mL).

African-Americans and those who have a father or brother with prostate cancer are considered to be at higher risk for the disease.

Men who have prostate cancer often have reduced free PSA. If total PSA is only slightly increased, testing for free PSA may be necessary. If the ratio of free PSA to total PSA is less than 25%, cancer may be present, and needle biopsy of the prostate gland may be necessary.

FOLLOW-UP: Any elevation of PSA requires consultation with a physician or a surgeon specializing in Urology. Whether immediate treatment or "watchful waiting" is the best course of action is a difficult decision that has to be made by the patient after he has been made aware of the various choices of therapy and the possible complications and consequences of each. The age of the patient at the time the disease is diagnosed, as well as the size of the tumor and whether it is localized or has spread to other parts of the body are important factors that must be discussed at length and in detail with a physician, and with his family before a decision is made concerning what treatment—if any—is best.

7. RANDOM BLOOD SUGAR

TYPICAL WORRY: *My urinalysis showed sugar. My doctor told me to have a blood test done to find out if I have diabetes.*

TEST: Random Blood Glucose ("Sugar") Test

TEST RESULT: (*example*) 256 mg/dL (SI: 8.7 mmol/L)

URGENCY LEVEL: Action: __√__ Decision: _____

NORMAL RANGE: Adult (non-pregnant): < 200 mg/dL (SI: <11.2 mmol/L)

ORIGIN OR SOURCE OF SUBSTANCES TESTED FOR: glucose (sugar) in a blood or plasma sample.

DIFFERENTIAL DIAGNOSIS:

If test results are HIGH, >200 mg/dL (SI: >11.2 mmol/L) or higher:

   impairment of glucose tolerance
   diabetes mellitus
   drug (such as a diuretic or a corticoid) effect
   severe liver disease
   alcoholism;

If test results are LOW, < 50 mg/dL (SI: < 2.8 mmol/L):

   a diabetic who has injected too much insulin
   pancreatic or other tumors
   liver disease
   malnutrition (e.g., anorexia nervosa) or starvation
   hormonal disorder related to the adrenal or pituitary gland.

COMMENT: Sugar is synonymous with glucose in the blood. Because it is often inconvenient or difficult to have a blood sugar test done after the necessary eight hours of fasting required for a Fasting Blood Sugar (FBS), most blood sugar tests are done *randomly* and are referred to as Random Blood Sugar. Fasting Blood Sugar test values are usually quite different from Random Blood Sugar test results. Any HIGH blood sugar results should be retested after fasting for eight hours, or done as a 2 hour Post-prandial (i.e., after eating) Blood Glucose test, or by a Glucose Tolerance Test (*see Chapter 15, "GTT"*).

A high-risk individual—one who is overweight, has an HDL cholesterol below 35 mg/dL (SI: < 0.9 mmol/L), a triglyceride level above 250 mg/dL (SI: 2.8 mmol/L), has a close relative with diabetes, had a baby that weighed more than 9 pounds at birth, or had a borderline normal blood sugar test result on a previous testing—should have blood sugar tests annually. Diabetics should monitor their treatment program results periodically by having a Hemoglobin A1c test done (*see Chapter 15, "Hb A1c"*) which will indicate how well blood sugar levels have been controlled in the previous three months.

FOLLOW-UP: Call or see your doctor if your test result is out of the normal range. Your physician may choose to do additional tests to rule out causes other than diabetes in the above Differential Diagnoses for your abnormal blood sugar test result. If your Hemoglobin A1c test result is higher than 65%, your blood sugar has not been optimally controlled.

8. THYROID STIMULATING HORMONE (TSH)

TYPICAL WORRY: *I'm tired all the time and I don't have the pep I used to have. Maybe I'm just getting old, or something's the matter with me.*

TEST: Thyroid stimulating hormone (TSH)

TEST RESULT: (*example*): TSH 5.3 mIU/L

URGENCY LEVEL: Action: __√__ Decision: _____

NORMAL RANGE: adults 20-55 yrs.:0.4-4.2 mIU/L, gradually increasing up to 10.0 mIU/L at age 80 or older.

ORIGIN OR SOURCE OF SUBSTANCES TESTED FOR: a hormone produced by the pituitary gland that affects the thyroid gland.

DIFFERENTIAL DIAGNOSIS:

If the TSH test result is HIGH:

> Hypothyroidism (too little thyroid hormone being produced).

If the TSH test result is LOW:

> Possibly hyperthyroidism (too much thyroid hormone being produced).

COMMENT: The TSH test replaces many older thyroid tests (e.g., BMR, T-4, T-3, etc.) used as screening tests. Very low values (>0.10 mIU/L) are panic values because of thyroid hormone's effect on the heart—causing an increased heart rate or an abnormal rhythym, especially in older patients (if you are drawing Social Security, you're an older patient!).

Hypothyroidism is often overlooked by members of the family and often even by doctors because it usually comes on very gradually and mimics the signs of senility and depression. TSH is an important screening test in the annual check-up in an elderly person.

There is an old medical aphorism ("saying"): "You can only diagnose something that you have thought of." The TSH test is often overlooked by practicioners in ordering a battery (group) of annual check-up screening tests, especially for elderly patients, and so Grandma's or Grandpa's debilitating but treatable hypothyroidism often goes unsuspected, undiagnosed, and untreated.

FOLLOW-UP: If laboratory tests suggest a thyroid disease or disorder, consult your physician. Thyroid medication (sometimes taken to lose weight) can be dangerous. Thyroid pills should *only* be taken under close medical supervision.

9. URINALYSIS WITH MICROSCOPIC EXAMINATION

TYPICAL WORRY: *I have burning when I urinate, and my urine looks like it might have blood in it.*

TEST: Urinalysis with microscopic examination.

TEST RESULTS and NORMAL VALUES:

Test	Test Results (example)	Normal Values
Specific Gravity	1.026	1.003-1.029
pH	5.6	4.5-7.8
Protein	2+	Negative
Ketones	Negative	Negative
Glucose	2+	Negative
Bilirubin	Negative	Negative
Urobilinogen	Negative	0.1-1.0 EU*/dL
Leukocyte esterase	Positive	Negative
Nitrite	Positive	Negative
Occult blood	Positive	Negative
Bacteria	3+	Negative
RBC	120/hpf**	0-5/hpf
WBC	3+	0-5/hpf
Casts	Negative	Negative
Crystals	Calcium phosphate	Negative

* EU: Ehrlich unit ** hpf: high power field of microscopic magnification

URGENCY LEVEL: Action: _√_ Decision: _____

ORIGIN OR SOURCE OF SUBSTANCES TESTED FOR: a filtrate of blood produced by the kidneys.

DIFFERENTIAL DIAGNOSIS:

In this example, the presence of blood, protein, nitrite, leukocyte esterase, bacteria and calcium phosphate crystals suggests kidney stones and infection of the urine; the presence of glucose suggests the possibility of diabetes.

COMMENT: Urinalysis is the most inexpensive broad screening test that can be performed on body fluids, but when abnormalities are found they may be non-specific. The urine reflects many chemical reactions taking place in the body because it is a selective filtrate of the blood transporting various chemicals and enzymes. Any abnormality should be followed up in an attempt to find an underlying cause.

Many diseases such as those of the bladder and kidneys, diabetes, chemical imbalances reflecting hormonal problems, and urinary tract infections or malignancies are first detected because of abnormalities discovered by urinalysis. Too often these have gone undetected for long periods because the urine was not periodically examined and so important abnormalities or trends were not detected.

Strangely, urinalysis is often not ordered by physicians because it has been bureaucratically declared by some to be a cost-ineffective test. Its value in early disease detection far outweighs the small cost of performing the test.

FOLLOW-UP: Any abnormality in the Urinalysis should be brought to the attention of your healthcare provider for evaluation.

CHAPTER 13

Blood Disease Tests

1. Activated Partial Thromboplastin Time (APTT)

2. Cobalamin (Vitamin B_{12})

3. Complete Blood Count (CBC)

4. Folic Acid

5. Anemia, Red Cell Abnormalities and Polycythemia
   A. Blood loss anemia
   B. Bone marrow deficiency anemia
   C. Chronic Disease Anemia
   D. Hemolytic anemia
   E. Iron deficiency anemia
   F. Megaloblastic (Pernicious) anemia
   G. Nutritional anemia
   H. Polycythemia
   I. Sickle cell anemia

6. Lead

7. Prothrombin Time (PT)

8. Serum Iron

1. ACTIVATED PARTIAL THROMBOPLASTIN TIME (APTT)

TYPICAL WORRY: *I'm on heparin as a blood-thinner and now I have had several long nose bleeds. I wonder if my heparin dosage is right.*

TEST: Activated Partial Thromboplastin Time

TEST RESULT: *(example)* 50 seconds (SI: 50 seconds)

URGENCY LEVEL: Action: __√__ Decision: _____

NORMAL RANGE: 25-39 seconds (SI: 25-39 seconds)

ORIGIN OR SOURCE OF SUBSTANCE TESTED FOR: the patient's blood plasma, tested to discover specific blood clotting factor deficiencies as well as the effectiveness of an anticoagulant (blood thinner).

DIFFERENTIAL DIAGNOSIS:

If test results are HIGH:

> the dosage of the anticoagulant (heparin) may be too high, and bleeding may occur somewhere in the body.

If test results are LOW:

> the dosage of anticoagulant (heparin) is unlikely to lead to abnormal bleeding, but may be too low to be effective in preventing blood clots from forming.

COMMENT: If the test result is HIGH, the dosage may be at a level where acute internal or external bleeding is likely. If the test result is LOW, the dosage may be insufficient to prevent thrombosis (blood clotting in a blood vessel)—which is most likely the reason heparin was prescribed. The test is also used to identify deficiency of certain factors in the blood (there are many such factors) that might be causing abnormal bleeding problems such as black-and-blue areas in the skin.

FOLLOW-UP: If your test results are either HIGH *or* LOW (above or below the Normal Range), notify your doctor at once.

2. COBALAMIN (VITAMIN B$_{12}$)

TYPICAL WORRY: *I wonder if I need a shot of vitamin B$_{12}$ to pep me up.*

TEST: Cobalamin (vitamin B$_{12}$)

TEST RESULT: (*example*) 95 pg/mL (SI: 70 pmol/L)

URGENCY LEVEL: Action: __√__ Decision: _____

NORMAL RANGE: (*approximates*) 100-250 pg/mL
     (SI: 74-185 pmol/L)

ORIGIN OR SOURCE OF SUBSTANCES TESTED FOR: a vitamin of dietary origin (it is present in most multivitamin pills).

DIFFERENTIAL DIAGNOSIS:

If test results are HIGH:

> probably the result of dietary or injected vitamin B$_{12}$ and of little clinical significance;

If test results are LOW:

> pernicious anemia (but *only* if a patient has symptoms and physical signs suggesting anemia and test result fits in with other laboratory and clinical abnormalities); alcoholism.

COMMENT: The test is not specifically diagnostic of pernicious anemia, but rather an aid to the diagnosis. Low vitamin B$_{12}$ sometimes is a clue to the diagnosis of unsuspected chronic alcoholism. The results of a test for vitamin B_{12} are unreliable if the individual being tested is taking multivitamins or recently has had an injection of the vitamin. It is important to know that vitamin B_{12} does *not* give one "pep", or increased energy, although it is often given as a placebo to one of the worried well. Unless one is proven by testing to be vitamin B_{12} deficient, has pernicious anemia, or is an alcoholic with an associated dietary deficiency, there is no valid reason for an injection of vitamin B_{12} to be given. Every well-educated physician knows this; perhaps he or she may be knowingly using the injection of B_{12} as a placebo. *Caveat emptor!* ("let the buyer—patient!—beware!")

FOLLOW-UP: If you suspect you have anemia, contact your doctor for examination and several laboratory tests. These will be necessary to find out if you really are anemic, and if you are, to reveal the specific type of anemia you have so that the proper treatment can be started.

3. COMPLETE BLOOD COUNT (CBC)

TYPICAL WORRY: *My face is very red and my skin is pinker than it used to be.*

TEST: Complete Blood Count. This will include at least five tests:

> hemoglobin (Hb);
> hematocrit (percentage of the blood composed of red blood ce lls) (Hct);
> white blood cell (leukocyte) count (WBC);
> red blood cell (erythrocyte) count (RBC);
> platelet (thrombocyte) count (Plts).

Cell indices (MCV, MCH, MCHC, RDW) may also be included; these will be meaningful and important to your doctor if the Hb, Hct, or RBC (or all three) are abnormal.

A Blood Smear Review with WBC differential (the percentage of various types of leukocytes in the blood) is often also included.

TEST RESULTS: *(example)*

> Hb : 17.3 gm/L (SI: 0.93 gm/L)
> Hct : 53%
> RBC : 6,765,000 /cu mm (SI: 6,765,000 x10^{12}/L)
> WBC : 3,750 /cu mm (SI: 3.75x10^9 /L)
> Plt : 112,000/cu mm (SI: 112,000 x10^9/L)
> Smear Review:
> WBC differential: WNL;
> RBC : normocytic and normochromic;
> Plts: decreased.

URGENCY LEVEL: Action: __√__ Decision: _____

NORMAL RANGES:

Hb: (*female*) 12.7-14.7 gm/dL (SI: 127-147 g/L)
(*male*) 14.7 16. 7 gm/dL (SI: 147 167 g/L)
Hct: (*adult female*) 38-44 %
(*adult male*) 43-49%
RBC: (*female*) 3.5-5.0 10^6/cu mm (SI: 3.5-5.0 x 10^{12}/L)
(*male*) 4.3-5.9 10^6/cu mm (SI: 4.3-5.9 x 10^{12}/L)
WBC: 3,200-9,800 /cu mm (SI: 3.2-9.8 x 10^9/L)
Plts: 150,000-450,000/cu mm (SI: 150-450 x 10^9/L)
Smear Review: "WNL"; "Normal"; "Unremarkable"

ORIGIN OR SOURCE OF SUBSTANCE TESTED FOR: blood cells produced in the body's hematopoietic (blood-producing) system, the bone marrow, spleen, thymus gland and lymph nodes.

DIFFERENTIAL DIAGNOSIS:

If test results are HIGH:

a. Hb, Hct and/or RBCs: polycythemia (too many red blood cells) may be present as a result of dehydration, or an overproduction of red blood cells by the bone marrow;

b. WBCs: may indicate an infection or inflammatory process, bone marrow disease, or leukemia (uncontrolled production of white blood cells by the hematopoietic organs);

c. Plts: thrombocythemia (over-production of thrombocytes in the bone marrow) with consequent thrombosis (stoppage of blood flow by a clot in a blood vessel), a common cause of stroke and heart attack, or artery blockage elsewhere in the body with serious consequences.

If test results are LOW:

for Hb, Hct, or RBC: anemia is present because of:

a. blood loss,
b. a failure of the bone marrow to produce enough, or normal, red blood cells,
c. an abnormal destruction of red blood cells in the body, or
d. a genetic abnormality (*see in this Chapter, Anemia, Red Blood Cell Abnormalities and Polycythemia*);

for WBCs: may indicate a viral infection or a bone marrow disorder;
for Plts: thrombocytopenia (under-production or loss of thrombocytes); may suggest a blood clotting disorder.

COMMENT: The WBC and Plt count in the CBC are unrelated to anemia in most instances. If the CBC does report these parts of the test to be abnormal as well as the RBC portions, there may be a serious bone marrow disorder. Not all laboratories include a Smear Review or Differential WBC, (the examination of a stained thin layer of blood under the microscope), or is automatically performed by a special laboratory instrument. The differential report includes the percentage of the different types of white blood cells in the blood sample: polymorpho—nuclear leukocytes (polys), lymphocytes (lymphs), monocytes (monos), eosinophils (eos), and basophils (basos) as well as thrombocytes (platelets).

Some laboratories may only perform the Smear Review on specific order by the doctor. Any significant abnormality in the Smear Review should be interpreted by a physician. The Smear Review is often omitted from the CBC because it is said to be "not cost-effective" (i.e., not enough "bang-for-the-buck" from an HMO's or insurance company's point of view) ; nevertheless, the blood smear may provide important information helpful in diagnosis (e.g., viral infections, parasite infestation, allergies, infectious mononucleosis, etc.).

Proper treatment of hematological diseases depends on finding the exact cause of the disease. For instance, not all anemias respond to iron medication, and only rarely (when pernicious anemia is diagnosed) are injections of vitamin B_{12} helpful; each of the many types of anemia requires treatment specific for the type of anemia diagnosed. (*See in Chapter 13, "Anemias, Red Blood Cell Abnormalities and Polycythemia" a broader discussion of various hematologic disorders revealed by abnormal test results in the CBC*).

FOLLOW-UP: See your doctor for evaluation of any abnormal test result in the CBC. He or she may order that the test be repeated, or initiate an investigation to find the specific cause for the abnormality. This may involve takinga variety of tests.

4. FOLIC ACID (FOLATE)

TYPICAL WORRY: *I want to get pregnant, and I've heard my baby could have birth defects if I don't have enough folic acid in my body early in my pregnancy.*

TEST: Folic acid (folate)

TEST RESULT: (*example*) 0.7 ng/mL (SI: 1.6 nmol/L)

URGENCY LEVEL: Action: __√__ Decision: _____

NORMAL RANGE: > 2 ng/mL (SI: > 4.5 nmol/L)

ORIGIN OR SOURCE OF SUBSTANCES TESTED FOR: a vitamin present in a wide variety of foods and included in most multivitamin pills.

DIFFERENTIAL DIAGNOSIS:

If the test result is HIGH:

> of little clinical significance.

If the test result is LOW:

> low dietary intake; megaloblastic anemia or macrocytic (pernicious) anemia; chronic alcoholism; Crohn's disease; intestinal malabsorption syndromes.

COMMENT: It has been reported that unsuspected folic acid deficiency is common in pregnancy (about 33%), and can be associated with serious adverse effects on the unborn baby. *Pregnant women or women contemplating pregnancy should take folic acid, especially in the early weeks (first trimester) of pregnancy.* Pernicious or megaloblastic anemia can be diagnosed only when the folic acid test result fits in with other laboratory and clinical abnormalities—the folic acid test alone is not specifically diagnostic of anemia of this type.

FOLLOW-UP: Call or see your doctor, who may order other tests to make a specific diagnosis; an example of such diagnosis might be dietary deficiency associated with chronic alcoholism.

5. ANEMIA, RED BLOOD CELL ABNORMALITIES, AND POLYCYTHEMIA

There are several commonly occurring types of anemias. There are also *hemoglobinopathies*: diseases of the body genetically transmitted that are reflected in abnormalities in the red cells of the blood and consequently causing anemia. *Polycythemia* is reflected in a too-high level of red blood cells in the blood.

A few laboratory tests are helpful in sorting out the various anemias, the hemoglobinopathies, and polycythemia. These tests are for:

Hemoglobin (Hb)

Hematocrit (Hct)

Mean corpuscular volume (MCV)

Mean corpuscular hemoglobin (MCH)

Mean corpuscular hemoglobin concentration (MCHC)

Hemoglobin electrophoresis (separates several genetically transmitted abnormalities of the hemoglobin molecule in the red blood cell).

Bone marrow aspiration and biopsy.

Information about the meaning of several common blood disease test result combinations, the causes of test result abnormalities, some symptoms and signs associated with these abnormalities, as well as suggestions for follow-up by a patient having anemia associated with these red blood cell abnormalities are included here. Each type of anemia requires different treatment; therefore it is essential that the type of anemia be identified. The same is true of polycthemia, which exists in two forms which need to be identified, the *acute* and the *vera* (chronic) form.

A. BLOOD-LOSS ANEMIA
Typical test results:

Hb: LOW
MCV: NORMAL (or LOW if blood loss is chronic)
MCH: NORMAL (or LOW if blood loss is chronic)

The cause: blood is escaping from the body faster than the bone marrow can produce replacement. This can occur following bleeding from wounds, severe internal organ injury (such as a torn liver or spleen in an auto accident), stomach ulcers, cancer of the uterus, kidneys, bladder, or gastro-intestinal tract, following delivery of a baby, heavy menstrual blood loss, or a surgical procedure from which there is heavy blood loss.

Some of the frequently occurring symptoms or signs: shortness of breath; pallor; fatigue; weakness; obvious hemorrhage; blood in the urine; bloody or black stools.

Follow-up: see a physician, who may order: stool for occult blood; urinalysis; serum iron (SI); complete blood count (CBC).

B. BONE MARROW DISEASE
Typical Test results:

Hb: LOW
MCV: *usually* NORMAL
MCH: *usually* NORMAL

The cause: the bone marrow (where blood is formed) is not producing enough red blood cells to keep up with the normal wearing out of red blood cells (they last about 120 days). This may be due to a disease such as leukemia; a malignant tumor which has spread to the bone marrow and is crowding out the cells the marrow normally produces; a reaction to drugs as in chemotherapy; or due to lack of stimulating substance (erythropoietin, produced in the kidneys)which promotes the production of red blood cells.

Some of the frequently occuring symptoms or signs: pallor; weakness; fatigue; bone pain; shortness of breath.

Follow-up: see a physician, who may order: Stool for occult blood; urninalysis; serum iron (SI); complete blood count (CBC); colonoscopy.

C. CHRONIC DISEASE ANEMIA
Typical test results:

Hb: LOW
MCV: NORMAL
MCH: NORMAL

The cause: the body is responding to a persistent disease process by not producing enough red blood cells; the cause is not well understood. It may occur in patients with chronic debilitating diseases such as rheumatoid arthritis, kidney disease, a malignancy, or AIDS.

Some of the frequently occuring symptoms or signs: these depend on those of the underlying disease; pallor; shortness of breath, weakness, and fatigue are common.

Follow-up: see a physician, who may order tests appropriate for detection of the underlying disease: serum iron (SI); total iron binding capactiy (TIBC); complete blood count (CBC).

D. HEMOLYTIC ANEMIA
Typical test results:

Hb: LOW
MCV: LOW or NORMAL
MCHC: LOW or NORMAL

The cause: red blood cells are being destroyed in the body; this may be the result of a genetic abnormality a person is born with, a blood tranfusion reaction, reaction to toxic materials or drugs, infections, parasite infestations, or an Rh or ABO blood type incompatibility during pregnancy or during a blood transfusion

Some of the frequently occurring symptoms or signs: pallor; weakness; jaundice; low or no urine ouput; dark urine; shortness of breath.

Follow-up: see a physician, who may order: anti-human globulin test ("Coombs test"); fibrin split-products; urinary hemoglobin; blood group and type.

E. IRON DEFICIENCY ("MICROCYTIC") ANEMIA
Typical test results:

Hemoglobin (Hb): LOW
Mean corpuscular volume (MCV): LOW
Mean corpuscular hemoglobin (MCH): LOW

The cause: the iron stores in the body have been depleted; iron is necessary for the production of hemoglobin. Common causes of insufficient iron are: unrecognized bleeding into the gastro-intestinal tract or heavy menstrual blood loss; insufficient iron in the diet; or poor gastro-intestinal absorption of iron from the diet.

Some of the frequently occurring symptoms or signs: pallor; weakness; fatigue; shortness of breath; the RBCs in the blood smear are *microcytic* (smaller than normal).

Follow-up: see a physician, who may order: serum iron (SI); total iron-binding capacity (TIBC); stool for occult blood; urinalysis (UA); stomach fluid testing.

F. MEGALOBLASTIC ("PERNICIOUS"; "MACROCYTIC") ANEMIA
Typical test results:

Hb: LOW
MCV: HIGH
MCH: NORMAL

The cause: this is a disease in which the body is not producing normal red blood cells because of a lack of intake or body production of essential vitamins, an abnormality of a stomach secretion, or a combination of these. This disease also affects the nervous system.

Some of the frequently occurring symptoms or signs: shortness of breath; pallor; fatigue; weakness; weight loss secondary to unsupervised dieting; anorexia or bulimia.

Follow-up: see a physician, who may order: serum iron; total serum protein, Vitamin B_{12}; folic acid.

G. NUTRITIONAL ANEMIA
Typical test results:

Hb: LOW

MCV: LOW

MCH: LOW

The cause: the is not getting enough of the building blocks of normal red blood cells such as protien, iron or vitamins to make enough normal red blood cells; RBCs are microcytic.

Some of the frequently occurring symptoms and signs: shortness of breath; pallor; fatigue; weakness; weight loss secondary to unsupervised dieting; anorexia or bulemia.

Follow up: see a physician, who may order: serum iron; total serum; Vitamin B_{12}; folic acid.

H. POLYCYTHEMIA
Typical test results:

Hb: HIGH

Hct: HIGH

MCV: NORMAL

MCH: NORMAL

The cause: in *polycythemia vera* the bone marrow is producing too many red blood cells; in *acute polycythemia* the fluidity of the blood is altered by dehydration, hyperthermia, extensive burns of the body, or overdose or overuse of *diuretics* ("water pills"). Therefore polycythemia is neither a hemoglobinopathy nor an anemia, but rather a too-great concentration of normal red blood cells in the blood. Whether chronic or acute, in polycythemia the blood is thickened, giving it a tendency to clot easily within blood vessels, possibly precipitating a stroke or heart attack.

Some common symptoms or signs: ruddy complexion; stroke (a brain blood vessel stopped up by a blood clot); heart attack (a heart blood vessel stopped up by a blood clot); dehydration; hyperthermia; extensive body burns.

Follow-up: see a physician, who may order: complete blood count (CBC); platelet count; or bone marrow aspiration and biopsy if polycythemia vera is suspected.

I. SICKLE CELL ANEMIA and other HEMOGLOBINOPATHIES

The three more common hemoglobinopathies (disorders of the RBCs) in the U.S. are *sickle cell disease, Hemoglobin C disease*, and *thalassemia syndrome*. Sickle cell disease is found in Afro-Americans, where the incidence of occurrence is 8.5%. All three are serious medical diseases and causes of chronic anemia associated with other changes in the body.

The cause: abnormalities of the hemoglobin molecule within the red blood cell, causing either the destruction of the RBC within the body under certain circumstances (e.g., *sickle cell hemolysis, sickle cell crisis*), or inefficient *synthesis* (production) of the hemoglobin molecule in the bone marrow (e.g., *hemoglobin C disease*). These abnormalities are genetically transmitted, and can be identified in the laboratory by the *hemoglobin electrophoresis* test and by the appearance of abnormal RBC forms and an increased number of *reticulocytes* (newly formed RBCs from the bone marrow) in a patient's blood smear.

Typical Test Results:
Hb: LOW
Hct: LOW
Hb electrophoresis shows:
    Hb C = Hb C disease
    Hb S = Sickle cell anemia
    Hb A_2 = Thalassemia
Blood smear review:
    increased number of reticulocytes=Thalassemia
    Hb C crystals = Hb C disease
    target cells = Thalassemia
    sickle cells = Sickle cell anemia

Some of the frequently occurring symptoms or signs: pallor; weakness; fatigue; bone pain; shortness of breath.

Follow-up: diseases in this category of anemias require continuing medical supervision. While not presently curable because of their genetic origin, symptoms and signs of disease may be alleviated, and complications can usually be helped to provide more comfort, increased function, and extended longevity.

6. LEAD

TYPICAL WORRY: *I live in an old house and my baby eats everything.*

TEST: Lead (test done on serum from blood)

TEST RESULT: *example)* 37 mg/dL (SI: 1.8 mmol/L)

URGENCY LEVEL: Action: __√__ Decision: _____

NORMAL RANGE: less than (<) 10 mg/dL

ORIGIN OR SOURCE OF SUBSTANCE TESTED FOR: a chemical element found everywhere in industrial society: soil, air, dust, paint, drinking water, food, exhaust fumes, "moonshine", automobile batteries, many folk remedies.

DIFFERENTIAL DIAGNOSIS :

If blood Lead is HIGH:

lead poisoning (plumbism); mental retardation, and "failure to thrive" in infants and children.

If blood Lead is LOW:

of no significance.

COMMENT: Lead is often an unappreciated occupational and environmental hazard causing varying symptoms; toxicity is rarely suspected (and thus infrequently tested for except in high-risk industries); *it is also an often unsuspected cause of retardation or "failure to thrive" in infants and children.* Minute old paint dust or chips may each contain thousands of micrograms (mg) of lead, and often are the source of lead toxicity. Industrial atmospheric pollutants containing lead are an increasing hazard to health in many localities in the U.S. and other industrialized countries.

FOLLOW-UP: Elevated blood levels require searching for the source of the pollutant, as well as obtaining medical care immediately, especially when elevations are found in infants and children. Current advice is that infants and children should be checked for evidence of elevated blood (serum) lead levels *at least once a year* up to at least age five years to prevent or arrest serious irreversible consequences of lead poisoning, such as mental retardation.

7. PROTHROMBIN TIME (PT)

TYPICAL WORRY: *I have been taking my blood thinner for a long time because of my heart attack. I haven't had my pro-time checked in quite a while.*

TEST: Prothrombin time (PT) ("Pro-time")

TEST RESULTS: (*example*) Patient: 58 seconds
Control: 11.5 seconds

URGENCY LEVEL: Action: _√_ Decision: ____

SIGNIFICANT VALUES:

   Control range: 10-13 seconds
   Therapeutic range: 2 to 3 times Control
   Panic range: > 3 times Control

ORIGIN OR SOURCE OF SUBSTANCE TESTED FOR: clotting factors in the blood produced by the liver.

DIFFERENTIAL DIAGNOSIS:

If the results are ABOVE the therapeutic range (effective treatment level):

   possible overdose of the anticoagulant (blood-thinner).

if the results are BELOW the therapeutic range:

   possible insufficient anticoagulant in the blood to prevent abnormal blood clotting.

COMMENT: This is a simple and inexpensive test, widely used for many years as a means of monitoring the adequacy or inadequacy of levels of anticoagulants in the blood such as heparin, but especially when coumarin and warfarin are used over a long term. The test is run and reported in comparison to a normal control (blood from a patient or a substance not altered by the use of an anticoagulant). It is often used as part of an evaluation of a patient with symptoms or signs suggestive of a bleeding tendency.

FOLLOW-UP: See your doctor if test results are either HIGH or LOW. He or she may order that the test be repeated or your medication dosage and/or your schedule for taking the drugs adjusted.

8. SERUM IRON (SI)

TYPICAL WORRY: *I think I may have tired blood, like I saw in the ad on TV.*

TEST: Iron Panel: Serum Iron (SI), Ferritin, Transferrin (Total Iron Binding Capacity, "TIBC"), Transferrin Saturation.

TEST RESULTS :

Serum Iron: 23 ug/dL (SI: 4.1 mmol/L)
Ferritin: 201 ng/mL (SI: 201 mg/L)
Transferrin (TIBC): 470 mg/dL (SI: 4.7g/L)
Transferrin Saturation : 18% (SI: 18%).

URGENCY LEVEL: Action: Ö Decision:

NORMAL RANGE:

Serum Iron: 60-160 ug/dL (SI: 11-29 mmol/)L
Ferritin: 12-263 ng/mL (SI: 12-263 mg/mL)
Transferrin: 200-380 mg/dL (SI: 2.0-3.8 g/L)
Transferrin Saturation: 20-50%.

DIFFERENTIAL DIAGNOSIS:

Disease	Serum Iron	Transferrin (TIBC)	Transferrin Saturation
Iron deficiency	D	I	D
Hemolytic anemia	I	N or D	I

Disease	Serum Iron	Transferrin (TIBC)	Transferrin Saturation
Chronic disease anemia	D	N or D	N or D
Liver disease (acute)	I	I, N, or D	I
Hemochromatosis	I	D	I

Key: I = Increased; D = Decreased; N = Normal;

COMMENT: All of the above diseases showing Increased (I) or Decreased (D) test results require immediate follow-up. If test results are within the normal range, disease is unlikely. (*Transferrin* is synonymous with *Total Iron Binding Capacity*—TIBC).

Increased *ferritin* levels may be also associated with hyperthyroidism, and susceptibility to the acute respiratory distress syndrome (ARDS).

FOLLOW-UP: Call your doctor or other health care provider, who may order other tests to establish a specific diagnosis if your test results are Increased (I) or Decreased (D).

CHAPTER 14

Cancer Screening Tests

1. Carcinoembryonic Antigen (CEA)

2. Estrogen Receptor Assay-
Progesterone Receptor Assay (ERA-PRA)

3. Occult Blood in Stool (Hemoccultä)

4. Papanicalou Cytologic Smear for Cancer
of the Cervix, Uterus and Vagina ("Pap smear")

5. Prostate Specific Antigen (PSA)

6. Sputum Cytologic Smear for Lung Cancer
("Sputum smear")

1. CARCINOEMBRYONIC ANTIGEN (CEA)

TYPICAL WORRY: *I've had surgery for cancer of the colon and worry about it spreading to my liver.*

TEST: Carcinoembryonic antigen (CEA)

TEST RESULT: (*example*) 23 ng/mL (SI: 23 mg/L)

URGENCY LEVEL: Action: __√__ Decision: _____

NORMAL RANGE: Non-smoker: < 2.5 ng/mL (SI: < 2.5 mg/L)
Smoker: < 5.0 ng/mL (SI: < 5.0 mg/L)

ORIGIN OR SOURCE OF SUBSTANCES TESTED FOR: an antigenic protein in the blood (antigen: a protein or carbohydrate capable of stimulating an immune response in the body).

DIFFERENTIAL DIAGNOSIS:

If the test result is HIGH:

possible spread of a previously diagnosed cancer of the colon, small intestine, or stomach.

If the test result is LOW:

usually of no significance, although some patients may have spread of cancer even if the test result is within the normal range (*false-negative*).

COMMENT: CEA is regarded as a "tumor marker" that may become elevated in a wide variety of cancers, but is particularly useful in determining if gastrointestinal cancer has spread to other organs such as the liver. It is not generally used as a screening test to find out if cancer is present in a worried well person who has no symptoms or family history of cancer.

FOLLOW-UP: Your doctor will likely order further tests and treatment if the test result suggests spread of your cancer.

2. ESTROGEN AND PROGESTERONE RECEPTOR ASSAY (ERA-PRA)

TYPICAL WORRY: *I've had surgery for breast cancer in my left breast, and the pathology report includes an "ERA-PRA". I don't know what that means.*

TEST: Estrogen and progesterone receptor assay.

TEST RESULTS: (example) ERA: Positive; PRA: Positive

URGENCY LEVEL: Action: __√__ Decision: _____

DESIRABLE RESULTS: ERA and PRA are both "Positive" or "Strongly positive".

ORIGIN OR SOURCE OF SUBSTANCES TESTED FOR: breast tissue containing cancer cells.

DIFFERENTIAL DIAGNOSIS:

If ERA is POSITIVE and PRA is NEGATIVE:

> a good response to treatment with hormones is likely, but long term prognosis may be variable and unpredictable;

If both ERA and PRA are POSITIVE:

> a good response to hormonal treatment can be expected in 45% of premenopausal women and in over 60% of postmenopausal women; overall prognosis is usually favorable.

If ERA is NEGATIVE and PRA is POSITIVE:

> response of the cancer to hormones may be limited,
> but hormonal treatment is not useless

If both ERA and PRA are NEGATIVE:

> the cancer will probably be unresponsive, or only
> marginally responsive to hormonal treatment; overall
> prognosis is unpredictable.

COMMENT: This test is done on cancer tissue removed from the breast to determine whether the cancer may or may not be responsive to treatment with hormones. The ERA is the better predictor of response to hormonal treatment, but in some clinical studies PRA positivity has been shown to be better related to an overall prognosis, despite the apparent limited hormonal therapy response by the tumor. Hormone non-responsive tumors are usually more effectively treated with chemotherapy and other types of cancer treatment such as radiation. (*See Chapter 10, Surgical Pathology Biopsy Report for further discussion of breast cancer and its management in relation to the surgical pathology report.*)

FOLLOW-UP: Cancer treatment is a medical specialty (Oncology). Breast cancer patients are often placed on therapy protocols (treatment plans) by oncologists as part of long-term studies to determine the best methods of treatment in the future. Most physicians work closely with oncologists in the care and management of their patients with breast (and other) cancers, an often fickle and occasionally treacherous disease.

3. OCCULT BLOOD IN THE STOOL

TYPICAL WORRY: *I know cancer of the colon is common and my father died from it. I've never had a test to see if I might be getting it too.*

TEST: Guaic test for Occult (hidden) Blood

TEST RESULT: (*example*) Positive for occult blood.

URGENCY LEVEL: Action: __√__ Decision: _____

NORMAL RANGE: Negative for occult blood.

ORIGIN OR SOURCE OF SUBSTANCES TESTED FOR: Blood leaking into the esophagus or intestinal tract in an amount too small to be noticed in the stool (feces, shit).

DIFFERENTIAL DIAGNOSIS:

If the screening test or culture is POSITIVE:

> bleeding into the esophago-gastrointestinal tract (i.e., from the back of the mouth to the anus; it includes the esophagus, the stomach, the small intestine, the large intestine, rectum and anus).

If the screening test or culture is NEGATIVE:

> no bleeding into the esophago-gastrointestinal tract.

COMMENT: The test has *low specificity* and *low sensitivity (for what these terms mean, see Part I, Chapter 8),* so there are often *false-positives* and *false-negatives.* However, it is the simplest and least expensive screening test for sources of bleeding somewhere in the entire gastrointestinal tract. The bleeding could come from ulcers, polyps, cancer, or varicose veins at the gastroesophageal junction (where the sophagus connects with the stomach) that have ruptured. Test kits are available (e.g., Hemoccultä) for detecting small amounts of blood, and most frequently used as a screening test for colon cancer; kit instructions have to be followed carefully to avoid *false-positive* test results. Death from colon cancer is currently second only to lung cancer in the United States. Early detection can lead to proper treatment and often to complete cure by surgical removal of a cancer or a pre-cancerous polyp.

FOLLOW-UP: If blood is found in the stool, notify your doctor at once. Colonoscopy or other procedures often are necessary as an immediate first step in follow-up of a report of blood in the stool in order to rule out cancer of the colon or other lesions in the gastrointestinal tract.

4. PAPANICALOU CYTOLOGIC SMEAR FOR CANCER OF THE CERVIX, UTERUS AND VAGINA ("PAP SMEAR")

TYPICAL WORRY: *I haven't had a Pap Smear for many years, and I know I should, there's so much cancer around.*

TEST: Papanicalou Cytologic Test for Cancer of the Cervix, Uterus and Vagina.

TEST RESULT: (*example*) Atypical squamous cells of undetermined significance ("ASCUS").

URGENCY LEVEL: Action: __√__ Decision: _____

NORMAL RANGE: Normal smear ; WNL; No evidence of malignancy.

ORIGIN OR SOURCE OF SUBSTANCES TESTED FOR: cells lining the vagina, cervix and inside of the uterus, mixed with secretions.

DIFFERENTIAL DIAGNOSIS:

If the report is POSITIVE:

>   for *squamous cell carcinoma*: cancer of the cells covering the cervix or lining the vagina;
>   for *adenocarcinoma*: cancer of the cells lining the inside of the uterus or cervix;
>   for *carcinoma-in-situ* (CIS): localized squamous cell cancer of the cells covering the cervix or lining the vagina.

If the report is ASCUS, or *low-grade squamous intraepithelial lesion* (LSIL):

the cause is usually indeterminate, but may result from inflammation, having given birth recently, recent sexual intercourse, or menopause.

If the report is: NORMAL SMEAR; WNL; NO EVIDENCE OF MALIGNANCY:

no evidence of cancer in this one smear.

COMMENT: A history of having one or more episodes of sexually transmitted disease (STD), human papilloma virus infection, or having begun sexual intercourse early in adolescence all increase the susceptibility of the female to the development of cervical cancer.

FOLLOW-UP: Studies have shown that it may take up to 7 years for cancer to develop after a Pap report of ASCUS or LSIL, although some carcinomas develop far more rapidly. Your doctor may recommend colposcopy (an examination with an instrument that allows close visual inspection of the surface of the vagina and cervix) and biopsy of suspicious lesions as a next step in evaluation (*see Chapter 10, "Your Surgical Pathology Biopsy Report"*).

An example of a strategy for follow-up, related to the patient's age and menstrual status:

Post-menopausal: your doctor may prescribe estrogen cream and a repeat of the Pap test (smear) in several months. and then schedule you for yearly Pap tests. Some doctors will recommend proceeding with immediate biopsy.

Pre-menopausal and post-menopausal women on hormone replacement therapy (HRT): your doctor may order a repeat of the Pap smear every 4 to 6 months; if three consecutive smears are normal, your doctor might order that Pap smears be done yearly thereafter—although this is a decison to be made by you after obtaining your doctor's advice.

A POSITIVE or POSITIVE FOR MALIGNANCY report requires *immediate* action to establish a diagnosis by biopsy, followed by appropriate treatment.

5. PROSTATE SPECIFIC ANTIGEN (PSA)

TYPICAL WORRY: *My father and my brother have prostate cancer and so I'm really worried about prostate gland cancer.*

TEST: Total Prostate Specific Antigen (TPSA).

TEST RESULT: (*example*) *22.0* ng/mL

URGENCY LEVEL: Action: __√__ Decision: _____

NORMAL RANGE: Thresholds for possible further investigation:

Total PSA:
Age: 40's: 2.5 ng/mL
50's: 3.5 ng/mL
60's: 4.0 ng/mL
70+: less than (<) 6.5 ng/mL.

ORIGIN OR SOURCE OF SUBSTANCE TESTED FOR: a protein, including both bound and unbound-to-protein fractions (the latter referred to as "free PSA") produced only by cells in the prostate gland.

DIFFERENTIAL DIAGNOSIS:

If test results are HIGH:

cancer of the prostate gland;
benign prostatic hypertrophy (BPH);
inflammation of the prostate gland (prostatitis).

If test results are LOW:

> prostate cancer is unlikely (a small or localized
> cancer cannot be absolutely ruled out);
> post-prostatectomy, or after any other treatment (e.g.,
> radiation) for prostate cancer that has partially
> or completely destroyed the prostate gland;
> falsely low, due to drug therapy for benign (non-
> cancerous) enlargement of the prostate gland
> (BPH); (*see COMMENT following*).

COMMENT: Some studies have shown that seventy percent of men between the ages of 50 and 70 years have a PSA below 2.0 ng/mL. Low test results may be due to medication (e.g., Proscarä; Avodartä) for prostate enlargement; be sure your doctor is informed if you are taking these drugs.

The rate of change ("velocity") of the PSA over time is significant; an increase of 0.8 ng/mL/year over three years is evidence that cancer may be present even if the test results remain within the normal range. Although PSA testing is useful, there is an appreciable number of *false-negative* test results i.e., when the test result falls within the normal range (2.6-4.5 ng/mL) but undetected cancer is present; thus testing annually or every two years is reasonable.

Any rise of the PSA from post-treatment low levels may indicate persistence or recurrence of the cancer.

If the PSA testing is done soon after a digital rectal examination ("DRE") of the prostate gland, there may be further elevation of the test results, but usually only if the test result is markedly elevated to begin with (i.e., >20 ng/mL).

African-Americans and those who have a father or brother with prostate cancer are considered to be at higher risk for the disease.

Men who have prostate cancer often have reduced free PSA. If total PSA is only slightly increased, testing for free PSA may be necessary. If the ratio of free PSA to total PSA is less than 25%, cancer may be present, and needle biopsy of the prostate gland may be necessary.

FOLLOW-UP: Any elevation of PSA requires consultation with a physician or a surgeon specializing in Urology. Whether immediate treatment or "watchful waiting" is the best course of action is a difficult decision that has to be made by the patient after he has been made aware of the various choices of therapy and the possible complications and consequences of each. The age of the patient at the time the disease is diagnosed, as well as the size of the tumor and whether it is localized or has spread to other parts of the body are important factors that must be discussed at length and in detail with a physician, and with the patient's family before a decision is made concerning what treatment—if any—is best.

6. SPUTUM CYTOLOGIC SMEAR FOR LUNG CANCER

TYPICAL WORRY: *I've been a smoker for forty three years, and I have a smoker's cough. This morning I coughed up stuff with some red and brown streaks, like blood. Am I getting lung cancer?*

TEST: Papanicalou Cytologic Test for Cancer of the Lung (Sputum smear)

TEST RESULTS: (*example*) Positive for malignant cells.

URGENCY LEVEL: Action: _√_ Decision: _____

NORMAL RANGE: "No malignant cells identified", or "Negative for malignant cells".

ORIGIN OR SOURCE OF SUBSTANCE TESTED FOR: sputum containing cells from the respiratory tract (sinuses, throat, larynx, trachea, bronchi, lungs).

DIFFERENTIAL DIAGNOSIS:

If the report is POSITIVE for malignant cells:

> cancer of the lower respiratory tract (bronchi or lungs), mid-respiratory tract (trachea, larynx), or upper respiratory tract (throat, sinuses).

If the report is NEGATIVE for malignant cells:

> no evidence of cancer in this one specimen.

COMMENT: The sputum cytological test is only valid if the sputum is properly collected (i.e., it is an early-morning, first "deep cough" specimen). If there is blood in *any* sputum specimen, especially that of a smoker, and the cytological report on this first specimen is "Negative for malignant cells", it is essential that at least two other sputum specimens be collected on successive days and each examined cytologically.

Sputum cytological examination is also an aid to the discovery of a variety of often unsuspected or undiagnosed viral and fungal infections, infestations by parasites, certain allergies, as well as several infrequently occurring diseases.

FOLLOW-UP: If you have blood in your sputum, contact your doctor as soon as possible. He or she may order other tests to make a specific diagnosis. These may include X-rays of the chest in search of the source of the bleeding. The only hope of cure or control of respiratory tract cancer is early diagnosis. Smokers should have sputum cytology testing at least yearly, even if no sign of blood is ever coughed up. They should not wait for that ominous sign of serious disease to appear.

CHAPTER 15

Chronic Disease Tests

1. Anti—DNA Test for Systemic Lupus Erythematosus (SLE)

2. Antinuclear Antibody (ANA) for Systemic Lupus Erythematosus (SLE)

3. Arthritis Panel (Systemic Lupus Erythematosus, Rheumatoid Arthritis, Gout)

4. CD4/CD8 Lymphocyte Panel and Ratio

5. Chloride Sweat Test

6. Cystic Fibrosis (CF) DNA Panel

7. Glucose Tolerance Test

8. *H. pylori* Serologic Test

9. Hemoglobin A1c

10. HIV-1/HIV-2 Serology

11. Kidney Function Panel

12. Kidney Stone Analysis

13. Lead

14. L.E. Cells for Systemic Lupus
Erythematosus (SLE)

15. Liver Function Panel

16. Microalbuminuria

17. Osteocalcin

18. Random Blood Sugar

19. Rapid Plasma Reagin (RPR) Test for Syphilis

20. Rheumatoid Factor (RF) for Arthritis

21. Thyroxine (T-4)

22. Uric Acid

1. ANTI-DSDNA TEST FOR SYSTEMIC LUPUS ERYTHEMATOSUS (SLE)

TYPICAL WORRY: *I have aching joints all over, a red rash on my face, and I'm worried that I might have something serious.*

TEST: Anti-dsDNA for SLE.

TEST RESULT: (*example*) 225 units (SI: 225 units)

URGENCY LEVEL: Action: __√__ Decision: _____

NORMAL RANGE: < 70 units (SI: < 70 units) (*Normal Ranges vary amongst laboratories*).

ORIGIN OR SOURCE OF SUBSTANCE TESTED FOR: an autoantibody to double-stranded (ds) DNA (desoxyribonucleic acid) in the nuclei (message centers) of body cells.

DIFFERENTIAL DIAGNOSIS:

If test results are HIGH:

Systemic lupus erythematosus (SLE).

If test results are LOW, NEGATIVE, or NONE:

SLE is very unlikely.

COMMENT: The test is almost specific for SLE, but may be slightly positive ("borderline") in some rheumatic and liver diseases. The test is often used to follow the course of treatment and/or the improvement or worsening of the symptoms of SLE. (*This test is included in the Arthritis Panel of tests*).

FOLLOW-UP: See your doctor, who may order other blood and urine tests to further evaluate and confirm the Anti-dsDNA test result.

2. ANTI-NUCLEAR ANTIBODY (ANA) TEST FOR SLE

TYPICAL WORRY: *I have arthritis and have heard that "lupus" can be one of the causes.*

TEST: Anti-nuclear Antibody Test (ANA).

TEST RESULTS: (*example*) Positive; Pattern: *speckled.*

URGENCY LEVEL: Action: __√__ Decision: _____

NORMAL RANGE: Negative.

ORIGIN OF SUBSTANCE TESTED FOR: Antibodies to cells or parts of cells produced by the body against its own cells (autoantibodies).

DIFFERENTIAL DIAGNOSIS:

If the report is POSITIVE, and the Pattern is:

> *Homogeneous:* SLE or other rheumatic disease; drug—induced antibody;
> *Speckled:* mixed connective tissue disease (MCTD); SLE; Sjorgen's syndrome;
> *Atypical speckled:* Scleroderma (a chronic skin disease);
> *Nucleolar:* SLE in a progressive stage (PSS).

If the report is NEGATIVE: SLE is unlikely.

COMMENT: Many drugs, as well as viral infections can cause a *false positive* ANA test. A few patients with SLE have a negative ANA test. (This test is included in the Arthritis Panel of tests.)

FOLLOW-UP: A POSITIVE test result requires evaluation by a physician.

3. ARTHRITIS PANEL

There are numerous diseases of which arthritis is a part, appearing as symptoms (pain, stiffness), or signs (swelling, redness). The more common diseases causing these symptoms and signs are: rheumatoid arthritis ("RA"), systemic lupus erythematosus ("SLE", "Lupus"), gouty arthritis, psoriatic arthritis (related to the skin disease psoriasis), and osteoarthritis. Tests for the first three of these diseases are included alphabetically in this Chapter:

> Systemic Lupus Erythematosus:
> *Anti-dsDNA Test for SLE*
> *Antinuclear Antibody Test for SLE*
> *LE cells for SLE*

> Rheumatoid Arthritis:
> *Rheumatoid Factor*

> Gouty Arthritis:
> *Uric Acid*

There is no specific laboratory test for the diagnosis of psoriasis. The arthritis associated with psoriasis (about 2% of patients with psoriatic skin lesions have arthritis) does not correlate well with the severity of the skin lesions. Uric acid may be elevated in some cases of psoriasis.

At the present time there is no laboratory test specific for osteoarthritis, a very common affliction of the elderly often diagnosable from the medical history, the characteristic appearance of the joints of the fingers on physical examination, and by X-ray of painful joints. Thus if lupus, rheumatoid disease and gout have been eliminated by laboratory testing and the skin lesions of psoriasis are not present, osteoarthritis is the likely "diagnosis of exclusion" in an older patient.

Other acute causes of arthritis include gonorrhea (*see Chapter 23, Sexually Transmitted Disease Tests: Urethral Culture and Vaginal Culture*), and rheumatic fever. For the arthritis associated with rheumatic fever, *see Chapter 11, Acute Disease Tests.* The Erythrocyte Sedimentation Rate (ESR) and C-Reactive Protein (CRP) are tests used to follow the progress of the inflammatory process but are not specific for the disease.

4. CD4/CD8 LYMPHOCYTE COUNT AND RATIO

TYPICAL WORRY: *I am HIV positive, and wonder if the treatment is helping.*

TEST: CD4/CD8 Lymphocyte Count and Ratio

TEST RESULTS: (*examples*)

> Total lymphocytes: 1250/cmm.
> CD4 lymphocytes: 325/cmm.
> CD8 lymphocytes: 425/cmm.
> CD4:CD8 ratio: 0.76

NORMAL RANGES:

> Total Lymphocytes: 1500-4000 /cmm. (SI: $1.5-4.0x10^9$)
> CD4: 450-1400/cmm (SI: $4.50-14.0x10^3$)
> CD 8: 190-725 /cmm (SI: $1.90-7.25x10^3$)
> CD4: CD8 ratio: 1.0-3.5

URGENCY LEVEL: Action: __√__ Decision: _____

ORIGIN OR SOURCE OF SUBSTANCE TESTED FOR:
Certain types of lymphocytes in the blood, separated by flow cytometry (a special laboratory test). The lymphocyte counts and ratios are indicators of immunodeficiency from *any* cause, including HIV infection.

DIFFERENTIAL DIAGNOSIS:

> If Total Lymphocytes are less than 1500/cmm, and/
> or CD4 Lymphocytes are less than 300/cmm, and/

or CD8 Lymphocytes are less than 190/cmm, and the CD4:CD8 ratio is <1.0, HIV is likely, and may be progressing to AIDS.

If Total Lymphocytes are greater than 1500/cmm, and/or CD4 Lymphocytes are greater than 300/cmm, and/or CD8 Lymphocytes are greater than 190/cmm, and the CD4:CD8 ratio is >1.0, HIV is less likely, or if previously diagnosed, is not yet progressing to AIDS.

COMMENT: The Total Lymphocyte count helps your doctor make decisions regarding treatment if you are HIV positive. If you are being treated and test results show abnormalities, your medication may have to be changed. AIDS (acquired immune deficiency syndrome) is a result of HIV infection but may take many months to develop. It has been observed that some individuals apparently develop immunodeficiency disease without known exposure to HIV, but this is quite infrequent.

FOLLOW-UP: Call your doctor if any or all of the above test results are abnormal. Your physician will choose the follow-up tests, if any, and any changes in medication that may be necessary.

5. CHLORIDE SWEAT TEST FOR CYSTIC FIBROSIS (CF)

TYPICAL WORRY: *I fear that my daughter may have cystic fibrosis because of our family history.*

TEST: Chloride Sweat Test

TEST RESULT: (*example*) 65 mmol/L (SI: 65 mmol/L)

URGENCY LEVEL: Action: __√__ Decision: _____

NORMAL RANGE: 0-40 mmol/L (SI: 0-40 mmol/L)

ORIGIN OR SOURCE OF SUBSTANCE TESTED FOR: chloride in the sweat excreted through the skin after application of a medication on the skin. (It is an *aid* in diagnosis Cystic Fibrosis, *not* a definitive test.)

DIFFERENTIAL DIAGNOSIS:

If the test results are HIGH:

> age 0-20 yrs: > 60 mmol/L (SI: same)
> adults: > 70 mmol/L (SI: same),then cystic fibrosis must be seriously considered, especially if CF symptoms exist.

If test results are LOW:

> cystic fibrosis cannot be excluded with certainty, but is unlikely.

COMMENT: This relatively inexpensive test is an aid in diagnosing CF, and is not a definitive test. Cystic fibrosis is likely if high sweat chloride is associated with foul-smelling stools, frequent bouts of pneumonia, chronic cough, (and in infants and children: failure to thrive, asthma, and frequent or severe gastrointestinal problems).

FOLLOW-UP: Call your doctor. Your physician will choose the tests, if any (*see 6. Cystic Fibrosis DNA Content, this Chapter*), that may be necessary to aid in the diagnosis of latent or overt cystic fibrosis. The Cystic Fibrosis DNA Content test is often recommended for pregnant women to determine whether or not they are genetic carriers for the disease. If both parents are carriers, the probability of cystic fibrosis in the child is higher than if neither, or only one parent is a carrier.

6. CYSTIC FIBROSIS (CF)
DNA CONTENT

TYPICAL WORRY: *My daughter has cystic fibrosis (CF), and I am pregnant again.*

TEST: Cystic Fibrosis DNA Content

TEST RESULTS: (*example*) "See Interpretive Report"

URGENCY LEVEL: Action: __√__ Decision: _____

NORMAL RANGE: 0-40 mmol/L (usual range: most laboratories dispense with giving a Normal Range, but rather issue an interpretive report).

ORIGIN OR SOURCE OF SUBSTANCE TESTED FOR:
A gene defect in the fetus, found in amniotic fluid during the 17th to 18th week of pregnancy.

DIFFERENTIAL DIAGNOSIS:

> Test results are highly specific for cystic fibrosis in the unborn fetus early in pregnancy *when test information is interpreted by a physician knowledgeable and experienced in genetic testing.*

COMMENT: The test is expensive, time consuming, and requires professional interpretation and counseling; the Cystic Fibrosis DNA Content test is recommended by many obstetricians for both parents if there is a family history of CF to determine whether or not they are carriers for the disease. If both parents are carriers, the probability of cystic fibrosis in the child is higher than if neither, or only one parent is a carrier.

An unsuspected carrier state for CF occasionally is discovered even when there is no known history of CF.

FOLLOW-UP: Call your doctor. Your physician will choose the follow-up tests, if any, that may be necessary, and will likely recommend appropriate genetic, social, and ethical counseling.

7. GLUCOSE TOLERANCE TEST (GTT)

TYPICAL WORRY: *I sometimes feel faint; I think I have low blood sugar.*

TEST: Glucose Tolerance Test (GTT).

TEST RESULTS: (*example*) Fasting: 63 mg/dL (SI: 3.5 mmol/L)

URGENCY LEVEL: Action: __√__ Decision: _____

NORMAL RANGE:

> Adult (non-pregnant female):
> fasting: 60-115 mg/dL (SI: 3.3-6.4 mmol/L)
> following drinking a standardized dose of glucose:
> > maximum rise after 1 hour: 184 mg/dL (SI: 10.1 mmol/L) maximum rise after 2 hours: 140 mg/dL (SI: 7.7 mmol/L)

ORIGIN OR SOURCE OF SUBSTANCE TESTED FOR: glucose (sugar) in the blood.

DIFFERENTIAL DIAGNOSIS:

If test results are HIGH (*impaired or decreased* glucose tolerance):

> diabetes mellitus; hyperlipidemia; hyperthyroidism; drug effect (steriods, e.g., cortisone); severe liver disease; pregnancy.

If test results are LOW (*increased* glucose tolerance):

alcoholism; drug effect (too much insulin injected); hypothyroidism; hypo*para*thyroidism; pancreatic islet cell (the source of insulin production in the pancreas) tumor; liver disease; malnutrition or starvation; disorders of the adrenal or pituitary gland.

COMMENT: The GTT is difficult to interpret, and has been discarded by most physicians as a useful test. However, some physicians strongly believe that every pregnant woman should have a GTT between the 24th to 28th week of pregnancy, and if the results are abnormally high, further testing for diabetes should be undertaken after the pregnancy is completed. Any test result above 140 mg/dL should be repeated.

The GTT is sometimes ordered to try to find a reason for a patient's fainting spells, or to reassure patients who are convinced (usually without justification) that they are suffering from "low blood sugar" and therefore have "no energy". An energetic, slim female may have a glucose as low as 40 mg/dL (SI 2.2 mmol/L) and remain physiologically normal. The 5 hour glucose tolerance test (GTT5) has been discredited as a valid test for hypoglycemia (low blood sugar) and now is rarely used.

FOLLOW-UP: Call your doctor if you have fainting spells or other worrisome symptoms. The cause is almost always something other than "low blood sugar". A physician will be able to select the best tests to evaluate such symptoms.

CHAPTER 15

8. *Helicobacter Pylori (H. Pylori)*
SEROLOGIC TEST

TYPICAL WORRY: *I think I have a stomach ulcer.*

TEST: *H. pylori* serologic test.

TEST RESULT: (*example*) Positive.

URGENCY LEVEL: Action: _√_ Decision: _____

NORMAL RANGE: Negative.

ORIGIN OR SOURCE OF SUBSTANCE TESTED FOR: a
    bacterium present in the stomach and/or the
    duodenum; *H. pylori* (previously classified as
    Campylobacter pylori) infection produces antibodies
    through the body's immune system.

DIFFERENTIAL DIAGNOSIS:

If test results are POSITIVE:

    peptic ulcer of the stomach and/or the duodenum;
    chronic gastritis.

If test results are NEGATIVE:

    peptic ulcer is unlikely but cannot be completely
    ruled out.

COMMENT: A breath test (UBT) for evidence of *H. pylori*
    that can be done in a doctor's office is also available
    and may be useful in testing children suspected to
    have an *H. pylori* infection. Bacterial culture of gastric

juice and surgical biopsy are also methods of identifying the presence of the bacterium in adults. There is a very high correlation between the presence of *H. pylori* in the stomach (and/or duodenum) with peptic ulcer and gastritis. There is an increased incidence of cancer of the stomach in patients with *H. pylori* infection.

The prognosis for ulcers associated with the presence of *H. pylori* is favorable; ulcers and gastritis are treatable with appropriate antibiotics and other medications.

FOLLOW-UP: If your test results are POSITIVE, see your physician. Your physician will choose the follow-up tests, if any, that may be necessary.

9. HEMOGLOBIN A1c

TYPICAL WORRY: *I'm a diabetic and I wonder if my blood sugar is under control.*

TEST: Glycated (glycolated) hemoglobin (Hb A1c).

TEST RESULT: (*example*) 11.0 %

URGENCY LEVEL: Action: __√__ Decision: _____

NORMAL RANGE: 4%-5.5%

ORIGIN OR SOURCE OF SUBSTANCE TESTED FOR: a form of hemoglobin in red blood cells that binds glucose to protein.

DIFFERENTIAL DIAGNOSIS:

If test result is HIGH:

> diabetes has not been under good control in the recent past (weeks or months).

If test result is LOW:

> diabetes has been under good control in the recent past.

COMMENT: When diabetes is not properly controlled by diet and insulin, complications of diabetes such as kidney damage, hypertension, and damage to the retina of the eyes can occur relatively quickly. Type I diabetics (insulin dependent, "IDDM") should have the test performed routinely every 3-4 months, Type II diabetics (non-insulin dependent, "NIDDM"), every 6 months.

FOLLOW-UP: Call your doctor, who may order other tests and/or adjust your insulin and your dietary instructions.

10. HIV-1/HIV-2 SEROLOGY

TYPICAL WORRY: *I'm afraid I've been exposed to HIV infection.*

TEST: Serologic test for Human Immunodeficiency Viruses (HIV-1 and HIV-2).

TEST RESULT: (*example*) Positive

URGENCY LEVEL: Action: __√__ Decision: _____

NORMAL RANGE: Negative.

ORIGIN OR SOURCE OF SUBSTANCE TESTED FOR: antibodies produced by the body's immune system in response to the HIV infection.

DIFFERENTIAL DIAGNOSIS:

if test results are POSITIVE:

> HIV infection is highly likely, but must be confirmed by a follow-up test (i.e., Western Blot test).

if test results are NEGATIVE:

> infection by HIV is unlikely, but early after exposure the test may be a *false-negative.*

COMMENT: Most, but not necessarily all diseases associated with this test abnormality are HIV-1 or HIV-2 infections, with or without AIDS (*A*cquired *I*mmuno*d*eficiency *S*yndrome). The prognosis is better for long time survival if treatment is initiated early.

Important: If the HIV test is negative after the presumed possibility of exposure, repeating the test in 2 or 3 weeks is essential, because the antibodies to the HIV virus may not yet have been developed by the body's immune system, even though the virus is present and active in the body.

FOLLOW-UP: If your test results are positive, see your physician immediately. Your physician will choose the follow-up tests that may be necessary, including test for other STDs. Advise your sexual partner(s) at once of your HIV infection if your HIV test result is POSITIVE!

11. KIDNEY FUNCTION PANEL

TYPICAL WORRY: *There's a family history of kidney disease, and I'm a diabetic and know diabetics often end up with kidney problems.*

TESTS: Blood Urea Nitrogen (BUN); Creatinine; Creatinine Clearance; Urinalysis with Microscopic Examination.

TEST RESULTS: (*example*)

> BUN: 42 mg/dL
> Creatinine: 2.5 mg/dL
> Creatinine Clearance: 25 mL/minute
> Urinalysis with micro: albumin ++
>   glucose +++
>   micro: WNL.

URGENCY LEVEL: Action: __√__ Decision: _____

NORMAL RANGE:

> BUN: 5-20 mg/dL (SI: 1.8-7.1 mmol/L)
> Creatinine: 0.3-1.2 mg/dL (SI: 26.5-106 mmol/L
> Creatinine Clearance: 75-125 mL/minute
> Urinalysis with micro: Normal urine (WNL).

ORIGIN OR SOURCE OF SUBSTANCES TESTED FOR:

> BUN: urea, produced in the liver;
> Creatinine: a chemical produced in the liver and
>   found in muscle, urine, and blood;

Creatinine Clearance: a measurement of how quickly creatinine is cleared (removed) from the blood by the kidneys;

Urine: a filtrate of the blood passing through the kidneys (removal of chemicals unneeded by the body and excreted in the urine).

DIFFERENTIAL DIAGNOSIS:

If BUN and/or Creatinine are HIGH:

kidney disease; heart failure; enlarged prostate gland.

If Creatinine Clearance is HIGH:

the result of vigorous exercise; pregnancy.

If BUN is LOW:

malnutrition, severe liver disease, third trimester (last three months) of pregnancy.

If Creatinine is LOW:

liver disease; loss of muscle mass, as in a wasting disease (e.g., late stage of cancer); small body size.

If Creatinine Clearance is LOW:

advanced age; kidney disease.

If Urinalysis is ABNORMAL

urinary tract (kidneys, ureters, bladder, prostate gland, urethra), or metabolic disease (e.g., diabetes, gout). (*See Chapter 12, Urinalysis with Micro for more information about Urinalysis*).

COMMENT: In this example of test results there is evidence of kidney disease of a serious nature, especially since there is glucose and albumin in the urine, and the Creatinine Clearance is very slow. The Urinalysis includes component abnormalities which may be important evidence in making a decision concerning whether urinary tract disease is the problem, or if a metabolic disease (e.g., diabetes) is present, or both; it gives important clues also about which part of the urinary tract might be the source of trouble.

FOLLOW-UP: A physician should be consulted if any of the Kidney Panel Tests is more than marginally abnormal.

12. KIDNEY STONE ANALYSIS

TYPICAL WORRY: *I get kidney stones, but the last time I passed one they didn't have the stones analyzed, so I don't know how to prevent getting another stone.*

TEST: Renal calculus (kidney stone) analysis.

TEST RESULTS: (*examples*): see below.

URGENCY LEVEL: Action: __√__ Decision: _____

NORMAL RANGE: (Not applicable).

ORIGIN OR SOURCE OF SUBSTANCE TESTED FOR: chemical compounds (filtered from the blood by the kidneys), which crystallize into calculi (stones) in the urinary tract.

DIFFERENTIAL DIAGNOSIS:

If X-rays have shown a stone:

> *calcium plus phosphate* stones:
> hyper*para*thyroidism;
> *calcium oxalate* (most common stones):
> hyperthyroidism; underlying malignancy in the body; sarcoidosis; metabolic kidney disease;
> *magnesium-ammonium-phosphate ("struvite") stones:*
> infection in urinary tract;
> *cystine* stone:
> cystinuria (a metabolic disease).

If the X-rays of the kidneys, ureters and bladder fail to show the presence of a stone ("radiolucent stone"):

uric acid stones:
gout; possible underlying malignancy in the body.

COMMENT: When a stone gets stuck in one of the ureters (the narrow tubes connecting the kidneys to the bladder) severe one-sided back or flank pain occurs and usually there is blood in the urine. Kidney stones are very common in Americans, and in white males particularly. Recurrence rate is high. Heredity, urinary tract infections (UTIs), the presence of malignancy, metabolic disease (e.g., gout, cystinuria) and lifestyle all can be related to the development of kidney stones. Modification of diet as recommended by a physician, and increased water intake are two simple life-style changes that can help prevent recurrences in some instances.

FOLLOW UP: Further studies, including urine culture and a serum chemistry panel and urine chemistry panel are indicated when kidney stones have been found to be present; these will be usually ordered by your doctor. Prevention of recurrences often depends on such further testing and the uncovering of an underlying causative disease. If stones do recur, there are techniques (e.g., lithotripsy) that can destroy some stones and relieve pain without invasive surgery.

13. LEAD

TYPICAL WORRY: *I live in an old house and my baby eats everything.*

TEST: Lead (test done on serum from blood)

TEST RESULT: (*example*) 37 mg/dL (SI: 1.8 mmol/L)

URGENCY LEVEL: Action: __√__ Decision: _____

NORMAL RANGE: less than (<) 10 mg/dL

ORIGIN OR SOURCE OF SUBSTANCE TESTED FOR: a chemical element found everywhere in industrial society: soil, air, dust, paint, drinking water, food, exhaust fumes, "moonshine", automobile batteries, many folk remedies.

DIFFERENTIAL DIAGNOSIS:

If blood Lead is HIGH:

> lead poisoning (plumbism); mental retardation, and "failure to thrive" in infants and children.

If blood Lead is LOW:

> of no significance.

COMMENT: Lead is often an unappreciated occupational and environmental hazard causing varying symptoms; toxicity is rarely suspected (and thus infrequently tested for except in high-risk industries); *it is also an often unsuspected cause of retardation or "failure to thrive" in infants and children.* Minute old paint dust or chips may each contain thousands of micrograms (mg) of lead, and often are the source of lead toxicity. Industrial atmospheric pollutants containing lead are an increasing hazard to health in many localities in the U.S. and other industrialized countries.

FOLLOW-UP: Elevated blood levels require searching for the source of the pollutant, as well as obtaining medical care immediately, especially when elevations are found in infants and children. Current advice is that infants and children should be checked for evidence of elevated blood (serum) lead levels *at least once a year* up to at least age five years to prevent or arrest serious irreversible consequences of lead poisoning, such as mental retardation.

14. L.E. CELL TEST FOR SYSTEMIC LUPUS ERYTHEMATOSUS (SLE)

TYPICAL WORRY: *I have arthritis and I've heard that lupus can be one of the causes.*

TEST: L.E. Cell Test for Systemic Lupus Erythematosus.

TEST RESULTS: (*example*) Positive.

URGENCY LEVEL: Action: __√__ Decision: _____

NORMAL RANGE: Negative.

ORIGIN OR SOURCE OF SUBSTANCE TESTED FOR: Antibodies to cells or parts of cells produced by the body against its own cells.

DIFFERENTIAL DIAGNOSIS:

If the report is POSITIVE:

Systemic lupus erythematosus (SLE); "lupoid" hepatitis; other rheumatic diseases; drug-induced antibodies; *false-positive.*

If the report is NEGATIVE:

SLE not present; *false-negative.*

COMMENT: Many drugs as well as viral infections can cause a false-positive L.E. Cell test result. Although sometimes used as a screening test for SLE, the L.E. Cell test is relatively insensitive, and is now only rarely used because of the more accurate Anti-dsDNA Test for SLE test. A few patients who have proven SLE may have both a *false-negative* L.E. Cell test and a *false-negative* ANA test. (*This test is included in the Arthritis Panel in this Chapter*).

FOLLOW-UP: A POSITIVE test result requires clinical evaluation by a physician as well as further testing.

15. LIVER FUNCTION PANEL TESTS

TYPICAL WORRY: *I have a yellow tint in my eyeballs and I drink quite a lot. Am I getting cirrhosis of the liver?*

FREQUENTLY INCLUDED LIVER PANEL TESTS: Alkaline phosphatase (ALP), Alanine aminotransferase (ALT), Aspartate aminotransferase (AST), Direct (Conjugated) bilirubin, Ferritin, Gamma Glutamyl Transferase (GGT), Lactic dehydrogenase (LDH), Prothrombin Time (PT), Total bilirubin.

TEST RESULTS: (*examples*)

ALP: HIGH
ALT: HIGH
AST: HIGH
Direct bilirubin: HIGH
Ferritin: HIGH
GGT: HIGH
LDH: HIGH
PT: PROLONGED
Total Bilirubin: HIGH.

URGENCY LEVEL: Action: __√__ Decision: _____

NORMAL RANGES:

ALP: (*varies by test method used* and *age*)
ALT: (*varies by test method used*)
AST: (*varies by test method used*)
Direct Bilirubin: = *or* < 0.4 mg/dL
(SI: = or < 7.0 mmol/L)
Ferritin: *male:* 20-250 ng/mL (SI: 20-250 mg/L)
           female: 12-263 ng/mL (SI: 12-263 mg/L)

GGT: (*varies by test method used*)
LDH: < 200 units/L (SI: < 96 IU/L)
PT: 10-13 seconds (SI: same)
Total Bilirubin: 0.3-1.0 mg/dL (SI: 5-17 mmol/L)

ORIGIN OR SOURCE OF SUBSTANCE TESTED FOR: various enzymes and pigments originating in the liver and bone and circulating in the blood. (All of the above Liver Function Panel tests can be measured from a single blood sample).

DIFFERENTIAL DIAGNOSIS:

If *any* of the above tests are HIGH:

liver disease or liver damage is likely (*but see COMMENT below for significance of some specific liver panel tests*).

If all of the test results are LOW or NORMAL:

liver disease is unlikely. Low test results usually are of little or no importance when evaluating most liver function tests.

COMMENT: Liver disease is serious, and abnormal liver test results should not be dismissed lightly. Interpretation of liver function tests is complicated and often difficult, and requires a knowledgeable and skillful physician experienced in diagnosing and treating liver (hepatic) disease.

Gall bladder disease, cirrhosis, viral hepatitis, liver or pancreatic cancer, hemochromatosis, and alcoholism are some of the more common diseases causing abnormal liver function panel tests. (In this fictitious patient example, there is evidence of serious liver disease, especially since there is clinical evidence of jaundice, e.g., yellow eyeballs).

Unsuspected or unadmitted alcoholism is a common cause of liver function test abnormalities.

Patients with non-alcoholic fatty liver disease (NAFLD) may show few or no signs or symptoms of the illness; this serious problem is quite common, and has been related to over-use or overdose of acetominophen which is present in many over-the-counter (OTC) drugs used for pain relief. The liver function enzymes in this Liver Panel will be helpful in uncovering this and many other diseases of the liver.

Prothrombin Time (PT) is a particularly sensitive test for evidence of liver disease but it is often overlooked by physicians as an important Liver Function Test. Not all prolonged PTs are due to an improper dose of a blood-thinner (e.g., warfarin); liver disease may be the underlying culprit.

High ferritin levels may also be found in or associated with hyperthyroidism, as well as susceptibility to the acute respiratory distress syndrome (ARDS), a serious lung disease.

(*Note:* One enzyme, ALP occurs in two forms, *liver* ALP and *bone* ALP; these can be tested for separately. Bone origin ALP is is *not* a liver function test. It is normally elevated in pre-pubertal children due to their rapid bone growth. Bone ALP is a tumor marker for bone malignancies.)

FOLLOW UP: A physician should be consulted if any of the Liver Panel tests are more than marginally abnormal. Referral to an internist or an internist sub-specializing in liver disease (hepatologist) may be necessary to

establish a specific diagnosis. Anyone with a known
history of hepatitis B or hepatitis C, diabetes,
alcoholism, obesity, or NAFLD should have periodic
testing of liver enzymes.

If you are trying to lower your cholesterol by taking one of
the "statin" drugs, you should have liver enzymes
checked periodically: every 3-6 months.

16. MICROALBUMINURIA

TYPICAL WORRY: *I'm a diabetic, and my doctor has told me that there is a test that will tell if my kidneys are going bad.*

TEST: Microalbuminuria

TEST RESULTS: (*example*) 42 mg/L albumin in urine (SI: 0.042 g/L)

URGENCY LEVEL: Action: __√__ Decision: _____

NORMAL RANGE: < 20 mg/L albumin in urine (SI: < 0.02 g/L)

ORIGIN OR SOURCE OF SUBSTANCES TESTED FOR: urine test for albumin in the blood that has leaked through the kidneys and has accumulated in all the urine that has been collected and saved over a period of 24 hours.

DIFFERENTIAL DIAGNOSIS:

If the test result is HIGH:

> diabetic nephropathy (disease of the kidneys) as a complication of:
>> diabetes mellitus
>> lupus erythematosus
>> hypertension (high blood pressure)
>> other acute or chronic kidney diseases.

If the test result is LOW:

> no evidence of kidney damage with this test.

COMMENT: Diabetes is very common in Americans (perhaps 12 or 13 million are afflicted) and kidney damage can occur in both Type I diabetes (insulin-dependent, "IDDM") and Type II diabetes (non-insulin dependent, "NIDDM") if blood sugar levels are not very closely monitored and controlled by diet and medication. The presence of albumin in excessive amounts in the urine is evidence of damage to the filtering apparatus in the kidneys, and once this has occurred, further damage may be arrested but existing damage is unlikely to be reversed. High blood pressure, SLE, and other disease of the kidneys must also be ruled out when microalbuminuria is found whether or not the patient has diabetes.

FOLLOW-UP: Call or see your doctor, who may begin a number of tests to identify the cause of the leakage of albumin (*see Kidney Function Panel and tests for SLE in this Chapter*). If diabetes is present, it must be very tightly controlled to prevent renal (kidney) damage.

17. OSTEOCALCIN

TYPICAL WORRY: *I'm past the menopause and have heard that if you have osteoporosis, it is easier to break a hip if you fall. Is there a test for osteoporosis?*

TEST: Serum Osteocalcin.

TEST RESULT: (*example*) 27 ng/mL (SI: 27 mg/L)

URGENCY LEVEL: Action: _√_ Decision: _____

NORMAL RANGE: female:

premenopausal: 0.4-8.0 ng/mL (SI: 0.4-8.0 mg/L)
postmenopausal: 3.0-12.0 ng/mL (SI: 3.0-12.0 mg/L)
male: 3.0-13 ng/mL (SI: 3.0-13.0 mg/L)

ORIGIN OR SOURCE OF SUBSTANCE TESTED FOR: a bone protein that is a sensitive indicator of bone metabolism.

DIFFERENTIAL DIAGNOSIS:

If Osteocalcin is HIGH:

osteoporosis is likely to be present.

If Osteocalcin is LOW:

osteoporosis less likely; possible response to treatment.

COMMENT: Osteoporosis (thinning of the bone), occurs in both men and women with aging. X-ray is an alternative way to test for bone density, a means of showing evidence of osteoporosis. Because women generally have smaller, less dense bones, they more easily break than those of men, and especially after menopause. Fractures of the hip are common in the elderly, and although surgical repair is often easily accomplished, complications lead to a high overall mortality in elderly women and men (in some reports as high as 10-30%). Osteoporosis is usually a treatable, if not a curable problem.

FOLLOW-UP: If Osteocalcin is high, see your doctor, who may order that the test be repeated, initiate an investigation into the cause of the osteoporosis, or initiate treatment by estrogen or other medication.

18. RANDOM BLOOD SUGAR

TYPICAL WORRY: *My urinalysis showed sugar. My doctor told me to have a blood test done to find out if I have diabetes.*

TEST: Random Blood Sugar (Glucose) Test

TEST RESULT: (*example*) 256 mg/dL (SI: 8.7 mmol/L)

URGENCY LEVEL: Action: __√__ Decision: _____

NORMAL RANGE: Adult (not pregnant): < 200 mg/dL (SI: <11.2 mmol/L)

ORIGIN OR SOURCE OF SUBSTANCES TESTED FOR: glucose (sugar) in a blood or plasma sample.

DIFFERENTIAL DIAGNOSIS:

If test results are HIGH, >200 mg/dL (SI: >11.1 mmol/L) impairment of glucose tolerance, because of:

> diabetes mellitus
> non-fasting specimen
> drug (e.g., diuretic or corticoid) effect
> severe liver disease

If test results are LOW, < 50 mg/dL (SI: < 2.8 mmol/L):

> a diabetic who has injected too much insulin
> pancreatic or other tumors
> liver disease
> malnutrition (e.g., anorexia nervosa) or starvation
> hormonal disorder related to the adrenal or pituitary
>   gland.

COMMENT: Sugar is synonymous with glucose in the blood. Because it is often inconvenient or difficult to have a blood sugar test done after the necessary eight hours of fasting required for a Fasting Blood Sugar (FBS), most blood sugar tests are done without fasting (*randomly*) and are referred to as Random Blood Sugar. *Fasting* Blood Sugar test values are usually quite different from *Random* Blood Sugar test results. Any HIGH blood sugar result should be retested after fasting for eight hours, or done as a 2 hour post-prandial (i.e., after eating) Blood Sugar test, or by a Glucose Tolerance Test (*see Chapter 15, GTT*).

A high-risk individual—overweight, has an HDL cholesterol below 35 mg/dL (SI: < 0.9 mmol/L), a triglyceride level above 250 mg/dL (SI: 2.8 mmol/L), has a close relative with diabetes, had a baby that weighed more than 9 pounds at birth, or had a borderline-normal Blood Sugar test result on a previous testing—should have Blood Sugar tests annually. Diabetics should monitor their treatment program results periodically by having a Hemoglobin A1c test done (*see Chapter 15, Hemoglobin A1c*) which will indicate how well blood sugar levels have been controlled in the previous three months.

FOLLOW-UP: Call or see your doctor if your test result is out of the normal range. Your physician may choose to do additional tests to rule out causes other than diabetes in the above Differential Diagnoses for your abnormal Blood Sugar test result. If you are diabetic and your Hemoglobin A1c test result is higher than 5.5%, your blood sugar has not been optimally controlled.

19. RAPID PLASMA REAGIN (RPR) TEST FOR SYPHILIS

TYPICAL WORRY: *I have been sexually active and I suspect my last partner may have a venereal disease.*

TEST: Rapid Plasma Reagin (RPR) Test for Syphilis.

RESULT: (*example*) Positive.

URGENCY LEVEL: Action: __√__ Decision: _____

NORMAL RANGE: Negative

ORIGIN OR SOURCE OF SUBSTANCE TESTED FOR: a substance produced by the body in response to syphilis and other infections.

DIFFERENTIAL DIAGNOSIS:

If the report is POSITIVE:

> syphilis; many *false-positive* reactions, including autoimmune diseases (e.g., rheumatoid arthritis; systemic lupus erythematosus); pregnancy; old age; viral infection (*e.g.*, infectious mononucleosis, hepatitis); drug addiction; parasitic diseases (e.g., malaria).

If the report is NEGATIVE:

> no disease; late stage of syphilis with anergy (failure to react in the test).

COMMENT: The test has very low specificity, but is more sensitive than a formerly-used screening test, the VDRL (Veneral Disease Research Laboratory) test. Many drugs and a wide variety of infections can cause a *false-positive* RPR test. A POSITIVE test for syphilis is a panic value in pregnancy. Syphilis is a treatable disease, especially in its early stages. A NEGATIVE test result does not necessarily mean that disease is not present; *false-negatives* can occur.

FOLLOW-UP: A POSITIVE test result requires immediate evaluation by a physician and a follow-up test, usually FTA-ABS. A patient who has one Sexually Transmitted Disease (STD) can have others at the same time, so a search for other STDs, (e.g., gonorrhea, HIV) that may also have been contracted must take place. This is necessary not only for the welfare of the patient, but also as a public health measure.

20. RHEUMATOID FACTOR (RF) FOR ARTHRITIS

TYPICAL WORRY: *I have stiff joints when I get up in the morning and I wonder if I might be getting arthritis.*

TEST: Rheumatoid Factor (RF).

TEST RESULT: (*example*) Positive.

URGENCY LEVEL: Action: __√__ Decision: _____

NORMAL RANGE: Negative.

ORIGIN OR SOURCE OF SUBSTANCE TESTED FOR: Antibodies produced by the body against some of its own proteins as an abnormal immune reaction.

DIFFERENTIAL DIAGNOSIS:

If the report is POSITIVE:

> one of many rheumatoid diseases may be present, (e.g., SLE) involving the connective tissues of the body, especially those tissues lining joints.

If the report is NEGATIVE:

> Rheumatoid Arthritis (RA) is not present; possible *false-negative.*

COMMENT: The test has low specificity and limited sensitivity. Many drugs, as well as viral infections can cause a *false-positive* RF test. As many as 20% of patients with rheumatoid arthritis and/or other connective tissue ("collagen") diseases may have a negative RF test result. Positive RF test results are helpful in the diagnosis of rheumatoid arthritis when combined with clinical findings supportive or indicative of that diagnosis. Other diseases, such as some sexually transmitted diseases (STD), Lyme Disease, and systemic lupus erythematosus (SLE) must be ruled out. (*This test is an Arthritis Panel test; see this Chapter.*)

FOLLOW UP: A POSITIVE test result requires evaluation by a physician. A NEGATIVE test result does not necessarily mean that disease is not present. Diagnosis will require a medical history and physical examination by a doctor.

21. THYROXINE (T-4; T$_4$)

TYPICAL WORRY: *I'm so hyper I can't even sleep.*

TEST: Thyroxine (T$_4$)

TEST RESULT: (*example*) 23.0 mg/dL (SI: 297 nmol/L)

URGENCY LEVEL: Action: _√_ Decision: _____

NORMAL RANGE: 5.8-11.0 mg/dL (SI: 75-142 nmol/L)

ORIGIN OR SOURCE OF SUBSTANCE TESTED FOR: hormone (thyroxine) produced by the thyroid gland.

DIFFERENTIAL DIAGNOSIS:

If test result is HIGH:

> hyperthyroidism; thyrotoxicosis with "thyroid storm"; Graves disease; goiter (enlarged thyroid gland).

If test result is LOW:

> hypothyroidism; myxedema.

COMMENT: The upper limit of the Normal Range for T$_4$ is higher in females on birth-control pills (BCP). A diagnosis of thyroid disease should not be made on test results alone; clinical information is essential to reaching a correct diagnosis. Some ill-advised individuals (often young and middle-aged women) take thyroid medication as a pep pill, for "crash" dieting, or for other reasons that are not always medically valid. Panic value ranges for this hormone are < 2.0 mg/dL) (myxedema coma), and > 20 mg/ dL (thyrotoxicosis); each of these diseases can be fatal if not treated.

FOLLOW-UP: If laboratory tests suggest a thyroid disease or disorder, consult your physician; thyroid medication should *only* be taken under medical supervision.

22. URIC ACID

TYPICAL WORRY: *I have a painful and swollen red big toe on my left foot. Could I have gout? I remember reading in Boswells "Johnson" that Dr. Johnson had a toe like mine when he had his gout attacks.*

TEST: Uric Acid

TEST RESULTS: (*example*) 18 mg/dL (SI: 1070 mmol/L)

URGENCY LEVEL: Action: _√_ Decision: ____

NORMAL RANGE: 2.0-7.0 mg/dL (SI: 120-420 mmol/L)

ORIGIN OR SOURCE OF SUBSTANCE TESTED FOR: a substance produced in the liver by the breakdown of protein in the body.

DIFFERENTIAL DIAGNOSIS:

If test results are HIGH:

>gout; gouty arthritis; kidney failure; lead poisoning; chemotherapy and/or radiation therapy; drug effects; hypothyroidism; hyper*para*thyroidism.

If test results are LOW:

>may be the result of taking drugs such as corticosteroids or aspirin in high doses; diabetics on insulin; malnutrition or diet low in protein; malignant tumors; kidney disease.

COMMENT: Relatively few individuals with higher than normal uric acid actually develop gout, but if one has symptoms of arthritis gout could be the cause and requires investigation by a physician. Lead poisoning (plumbism) is more common than is suspected; many physicians fail to think of it in their differential diagnosis, and a high uric acid may be the clue. Tumor-cell destruction is the cause of high uric acid in patients undergoing cancer treatment, and is to be expected. Uric acid kidney stones may occur as a result of high uric acid levels in the blood, and consequently end up in the urine (uric acid stones aren't visible on X-ray). Caffeine, theophylline and ascorbic acid (Vitamin C) may lower the serum uric acid test results, and you should tell your doctor if you are a heavy coffee drinker or you are taking these medications. (*This is an Arthritis Panel test; see this Chapter*).

FOLLOW-UP: If test results are high, medical consultation is in order. Your physician will choose the follow-up tests, if any, that may be necessary.

CHAPTER 16

Heart Disease Tests

1. Activated Partial Thromboplastin
   Time (APTT)

2. Cardiac Risk Assessment Test Panel
   Apolipoprotein A and B (Apo A and B)
   C-Reactive protein (CRP)
   HighDensity Lipoprotein Cholesterol (HDLC)
   Homocysteine (Urine cystine)
   Low Density Lipoprotein Cholesterol (LDLC)
   LDLC:HDLC ratio
   TC:HDLC ratio
   Total Cholesterol (TC)
   Triglycerides (TG)

3. Digoxn

4. Total Creatine Kinase (CK) and
   Creatine Kinase MB Fraction (CK-MB)

5. Troponin

1. ACTIVATED PARTIAL THROMBOPLASTIN TIME (APTT)

TYPICAL WORRY: *I'm on heparin as a blood-thinner and now I have had several prolonged nose bleeds. I wonder if my heparin dosage is right.*

TEST: Activated Partial Thromboplastin Time

TEST RESULTS: (*example*) 50 seconds (SI: 50 seconds)

URGENCY LEVEL: Action: _√_ Decision: ____

NORMAL RANGE: 25-39 seconds (SI: 25-39 seconds)

ORIGIN OR SOURCE OF SUBSTANCE TESTED FOR: blood plasma*.

DIFFERENTIAL DIAGNOSIS:

If test results are HIGH:

> the dosage of the anticoagulant (heparin) may be too high, and bleeding may occur somewhere in the body.

If test results are LOW:

> the dosage of anticoagulant (heparin) is unlikely to lead to abnormal bleeding.

COMMENT: Plasma is tested to discover specific blood clotting factor deficiencies in patients with bleeding tendencies, or to determine the effectiveness of anticoagulant therapy. If the test result is HIGH, anticoagulant dosage may be at a level where acute internal or external bleeding is likely. If the test result is LOW, the dosage may be insufficient to prevent thrombosis (blood clotting in a blood vessel)—which is likely the reason the anticoagulant (such as heparin) was prescribed.

FOLLOW-UP: If your test results are either HIGH *or* LOW (above or below the Normal Range), notify your doctor at once.

*   blood *plasma* consists of blood *serum* plus *clotting factors*; serum is what is left after red blood cells and cloting factors are removed from whole blood; neither plasma nor serum contain red blood cells.

2. CARDIAC RISK
ASSESSMENT TEST PANEL

TYPICAL WORRY: *My cholesterol is high. Am I going to have a heart attack?*

TEST: Blood lipoprotein panel, Urine cystine (homocysteine), and C-Reactive Protein (CRP).

TEST RESULTS: (*example is for a 45 year old female*)

> Total Cholesterol (TC): 255 mg/dL (SI: 6.6 mmol/L)
> HDL Cholesterol (HDLC): 32 mg/dL (SI: 0.83 mmol/L)
> LDL Cholesterol (LDLC): 163 mg/dL (SI: 4.2 mmol/L)
> Triglycerides (TG): 167 mg/dL (SI: 4.3 mmol/L)
> TC:HDLC ratio: 7.96
> LDLC:HDLC ratio: 5.09
> Apolipoprotein A (Apo A):155 mg/dL (SI: 1550 mg/L)
> Apolipoprotein B (Apo B): 130 mg/dL (SI: 1300 mg/L)
> Urine cystine (homocysteine): 76 mg cystine/g creatinine
> C-Reactive Protein (CPR): 27 mg/ml.

URGENCY LEVEL: Action: __√__ Decision: _____

NORMAL RANGES:

Cholesterol (TC) and Triglycerides (TG):

Age:	0-19	20-29	30-39	>39
TC mg/dL (SI):	155 (4.0)	175 (4.5)	195 (5.1)	210 (5.4)
(approximate HDLC mg/dL:	50 (1.3)	45 (1.2)	45 (1.2)	50 (1.3)
mean values) LDLC mg/dL:	95 (2.5)	110 (3.2)	130 (3.4)	145 (3.9)
TG mg/dL:	70 (1.8)	110 (3.2)	140 (3.6)	145 (3.9)

TC:HDLC: *male:* 3.4-9.5;   *female:* 3.3-6.9
LDHC:HDLC: *male:* 2.3-4.9;   *female:* 2.3-4.1

Apolipoproteins and Homocysteine:

Apo A: *male:* 80-150 mg/dL (SI: 800-1500 mg/L)
         female: 80-170 mg/dL (SI: 800-1700 mg/L)
Apo B: *male:* 50-125 mg/dL (SI: 500-1250 mg/L)
         female: 25-120 mg/dL (SI: 250-1200 mg/L)
Homocysteine: 40-60 mg cystine/g of reatinine

C-Reactive Protein:

CRP: < 8 mg/dL (SI: 80 mg/L); (when test is performed using low sensitivity tests such as agglutination or nephelometry);
<2 mg/dL (SI: 20 mg/L) (when test is performed using high sensitivity tests such as radioimmunoassay [RIA]).

ORIGIN OR SOURCE OF SUBSTANCES TESTED FOR: Substances produced by cells in the body and/or influenced by genetics, diet, exercise, alcohol intake, hormones, vitamins, medications; indolent low-grade infections (CRP).

DIFFERENTIAL DIAGNOSIS:

If Total Cholesterol and/or LDL Cholesterol are HIGH, there is a *higher* risk for coronary heart disease.

If HDL Cholesterol is HIGH, there is a *decreased* risk for coronary heart disease.

If Triglycerides are HIGH, there is *increased* risk for coronary artery disease (and stroke).

If APOlipoprotein and/or Cystine (homocysteine) test results are HIGH, either:

primary: hyperlipoproteinemia or homocysteine— mia (due to a genetic predisposition), or

secondary: hyperlipoproteinemia due to kidney disease; hypothyroidism; alcoholism; diabetes; obesity; lack of exercise; or *secondary* homocysteinemia due to lack of vitamins B_6, B_{12}, or folic acid; liver or kidney failure; postmenopause; use of drugs such as steroids, betablockers, thiazides.

If CPR is HIGH:

possible increased risk for coronary artery disease.

If HDL Cholesterol is LOW:

increased risk for coronary heart disease

If Apo A test result is LOW:

high risk of coronary heart disease;

If Apo B test result is LOW:

low risk of coronary heart disease

If *both* Apo A and Apo B results are LOW:

possible severe liver disease; malabsorption of dietary nutrients; malnutrition; hyperthyroidism;

If urinary Cystine (the test for homocysteine) is LOW:

probably of no clinical significance.

If CPR is LOW:

no significance.

Significance of TC:HDLC ratio:

Cardiac Risk Based on TC:HDLC Ratio

	Male	Female
1/2 average	3.4-4.9	3.3-4.3
Average	5.0-9.5	4.4-6.9
2 X average	9.6-23.	37.0-10.9
3 X average	>23.3	> 10.9

If LDLC:HDLC ratio is:

HIGH: *increased* risk for coronary heart disease.
LOW: *decreased* risk for coronary heart disease.

COMMENT: 1. All persons by the age of 20 should have their TC tested at least once *as a screening test* to detect any genetic predisposition to coronary artery disease, and every 5 years thereafter; those with abnormally high TC should have a Cardiac Risk Analysis performed to detect abnormalities early enough so that protective measures can be taken to prevent the development of coronary artery disease (CAD).

2. Antihypertensive medication (except calcium channel blockers) may have an indeterminate effect on test results.

3. Only some of the test results above may be abnormal; focus should be on any and every abnormal test result, even though many—or most—of the test results are within the normal range. It's the abnormal ones that count.

4. The TC:HDLC ratio and Apo A are considered to be valuable as indicators of cardiac risk; the Apo A:Apo B ratio is particularly useful as an indicator of coronary heart disease in young individuals.

5. Individuals with high TG and low HDLC are at higher risk for coronary artery disease and heart attack.

6. The table above is based on "average American" risk; however, American (defined here as one of those living in the affluent ambience of the United States) averages usually are higher than averages for many other ethnic groups worldwide. American averages would be considered abnormally high in

many, indeed most, other ethnic or geographically located populations.

7. CRP is an indicator of inflammation in the body, but does not tell where. Recent research has strongly suggested that the formation of obstructive plaques in the coronary (and other) arteries may be related to inflammation in the arterial wall. Elevation of CRP is thus another factor that should be considered in assessing cardiac risk and stroke. Preliminary data suggest that by treating the patient by encouraging loss of excess weight, more exercise, low-dose aspirin and "statin" drugs, a beneficial response would be reflected in reduced CRP levels.

8. Homocysteine is indirectly but reliably measurable by testing a 24 hour urine sample for cystine. It is now suspected to be as important a risk factor for heart attacks as are lipoproteins. Blood levels of homocysteine are strongly influenced by vitamins B_6, B_{12}, and folic acid; low levels of any or all of these vitamins may increase the levels of homocysteine in the blood and over extended periods of time may lead to development of atherosclerotic (fatty) plaques in the coronary arteries, and thus clogging them.

9. It has been recommended that homocysteine screening be performed on all infants, to uncover unsuspected primary (genetic) homocysteine abnormality because of its high potential for increased cardiac risk later in life.

10. Newer tests that have not yet gone through extensive clinical trials, e.g., "small LDL" and "HDL2B" may be found to be even better tests for cardiac risk than the tests discussed in this panel. Stay tuned.

FOLLOW-UP: Call your doctor when any of the above test results are outside of normal ranges; your doctor may order laboratory and other tests (e.g., Stress Test) to make a specific diagnosis. If your doctor has not ordered a CRP test and you are a moderate-to-high risk individual for coronary artery disease, ask your doctor to order it. If it is elevated, it should be repeated in 3 months for confirmation or to assay effect of any treatment or change in life style.

3. DIGOXIN

TYPICAL WORRY: *Is my digoxin pill dosage at the right level?*

TEST: Digoxin.

TEST RESULTS: (*example*) 2.9 ng/ml (SI: 3.7 mmol/l).

URGENCY LEVEL: Action: __√__ Decision: _____

THERAPEUTIC (EFFECTIVE) RANGE: 0.8-2.0 ng/ml (SI: 1.0-2.6 mmol/l).

ORIGIN OR SOURCE OF SUBSTANCE TESTED FOR: a drug that is used in the treatment of heart disease.

DIFFERENTIAL DIAGNOSIS:

If test results areHIGH:

> probably more digoxin in you blood than is necessary or desireable.

If test results are LOW:

> there may not be enough digoxin in your blood than your doctor intended.

COMMENT: Digoxin at a level higher or lower than your doctor has intended for your treatment should be corrected immediately, whether due to taking the wrong number of pills, too high a dose for your body to metabolize, or due to an incorrect prescription. Too high or too low levels often result from failure to take the medication on schedule, or perhaps because your prescription was not filled correctly at the pharmacy. The panic range for digoxin is > 3.0 ng/ml (SI: > 3.8 mmol/l).

FOLLOW-UP: Call your doctor immediately if your digoxin is out of therapeutic range; he or she will want to check your medication prescription and evaluate your heart condition.

4. TOTAL CREATINE KINASE (CK) AND MB FRACTION (CK-MB)

TYPICAL WORRY: *My husband had chest pain, and when we went to the Emergency Room at the hospital, the doctor ordered cardiac enzyme tests. What are those?*

TEST: Cardiac enzymes: Total creatine kinase (CK), and MB fraction (CK-MB)

TEST RESULTS: (*example*)   *Total CK CK-MB*
    2 hours after onset of chest pain: 200 U/L 15 U/L
    10 hours after onset of chest pain: 2250 U/L 215 U/L

URGENCY LEVEL: Action: _√_ Decision: _____

NORMAL RANGE: Total CK: (varies by method) immunoassay:

        males: 50-200 U/L
        females: 40-150 U/L
        CK-MB: < 6% of Total CK.

ORIGIN OR SOURCE OF SUBSTANCE TESTED FOR: Total CK: enzyme found in muscle, brain, and heart muscle; CK-MB: a fraction of CK enzyme found primarily in heart muscle.

DIFFERENTIAL DIAGNOSIS (CK and CK-MB):

If the report is HIGH after 6 hours and up to 72 hours:

    acute myocardial infarct (AMI or MI): injured or dead areas of heart muscle

If the report is NEGATIVE or LOW:

no evidence of cardiac muscle damage.

COMMENT: The CK-MB test has high specificity and sensitivity, but the time that the blood is drawn for the tests is critical. Many physicians order several tests over time after onset of symptoms of AMI (e.g., 1, 4, 6, 12, 24 hrs). A rapid rise in CK, and CK-MB as a percentage of Total CK is diagnostically confirmatory, especially when combined with a medical history, physical signs, and symptoms characteristic of AMI. Troponin (*see the next test in this Chapter, Troponin*) is increasingly used as another test for heart damage, but it is not reliable (may give *false-negative* result) until four hours after the onset of symptoms of a heart attack.

FOLLOW-UP: A significantly elevated CK-MB is a "panic value" that requires immediate evaluation, decision, and action by a physician. Follow-up testing will include electrocardiograms, cardiac telemonitoring, and admission to an Intensive Care or Cardiac unit where close observation of the patient is essential, and where cardiac support personnel and equipment are instantly available.

5. TROPONIN

TYPICAL WORRY: *My husband fell down and has chest pain, and I'm afraid he might have a heart attack. What tests will they do to find out if he has had a heart atack?*

TEST: Troponin

RESULT: (*example*) 1.25 ng/mL

URGENCY LEVEL: Action: __√__ Decision: _____

NORMAL RANGE: < 0.35 ng/mL

ORIGIN OR SOURCE OF SUBSTANCE TESTED FOR: a protein present in heart muscle fibers.

DIFFERENTIAL DIAGNOSIS:

If the report is HIGH:

> acute myocardial infarct (AMI or MI): injured or dead areas of heart muscle; severe chest trauma involving heart damage.

If the report is NEGATIVE or LOW:

> no evidence of cardiac muscle damage (*see COMMENT below re: timing of the test and possible false-negative*).

COMMENT: Troponin is a highly sensitive, very specific test for early damage to the heart muscle, whether it be due to chest trauma (as in an automobile crash injury) or due to a heart attack. It becomes diagnostic starting about four hours after the onset of symptoms, and remains increased for as long as a week after the heart muscle damage. Testing blood drawn shortly after the patient arrives in the Emergency Room, if less than four hours after the symptoms of a heart symptoms appear (e.g., severe chest pain), may not be positive, although heart muscle damage has indeed already occurred. A *false-negative* test result may result if the blood sample for the test was drawn sooner than four hours after the onset of symptoms. The CK and CK-MB test is often used along with Troponin in diagnosis and monitoring the progress of a patient's response to treatment (*see in this Chapter, Total Creatinine Kinase (CK)* and *MB Fraction (CK-MB)*.

FOLLOW-UP: A significantly elevated Troponin is a panic value that requires immediate evaluation, decision, and action by a physician. Follow-up testing will include electrocardiograms, cardiac telemonitoring, and admission to an Intensive Care or Cardiac unit where close observation of the patient is essential, and where cardiac support personnel and equipment are instantly available.

CHAPTER 17

Infant, Child and Adolescent Screening Tests

1. Lead

2. Phenylalanine (PKU) Test

3. Random Blood Glucose

4. Sexually Transmitted Disease (STD)

5. Total Cholesterol (TC)

1. LEAD

TYPICAL WORRY: *I live in an old house and my baby eats everything.*

TEST: Lead (test done on serum from blood)

TEST RESULTS: *(example)* 37 mg/dL (SI: 1.8 mmol/L)

URGENCY LEVEL: Action: __√__ Decision: _____

NORMAL RANGE: less than (<) 10 mg/dL (SI < 0.5 mmol/L)

ORIGIN OR SOURCE OF SUBSTANCE TESTED FOR: a chemical element found everywhere in industrial society: soil, air, dust, paint, drinking water, food, and automobile and truck exhaust fumes.

DIFFERENTIAL DIAGNOSIS:

If blood Lead is HIGH:

> lead poisoning (plumbism); mental retardation, and/ "failure to thrive" in infants and children.

If blood Lead is LOW:

> of no significance.

COMMENT: Lead is often an unappreciated occupational and environmental hazard causing varying symptoms; toxicity is rarely suspected (and thus infrequently tested for except in high-risk industries); *it is also an often unsuspected cause of retardation or "failure to thrive" in infants and children.* Minute old paint dust or chips may each contain thousands of micrograms (mg) of lead, and often are the source of lead toxicity. Industrial atmospheric pollutants containing lead are an increasing hazard to health in many localities in the U.S. and other industrialized countries.

FOLLOW-UP: Elevated blood levels require searching for the source of the pollutant, as well as obtaining medical care immediately, especially when elevations are found in infants and children. Current advice is that infants and children should be checked for evidence of elevated blood (serum) lead levels *at least once a year* up to age five years to prevent or arrest serious irreversible consequences of lead poisoning such as mental retardation.

2. PHENYLALANINE (PKU) TEST

TYPICAL WORRY: *I'm pregnant and I want my baby to be perfect!*

TEST: Phenylalanine (PKU).

TEST RESULTS: (*example*) 9 mg/dL (SI: 545 mmol/L).

URGENCY LEVEL: Action: _√_ Decision: _____

NORMAL RANGE: = or < 2 mg/dL (SI: = or < 121mmol/L).

ORIGIN OR SOURCE OF SUBSTANCES TESTED FOR: an
essential amino acid in the body necessary to build
proteins.

DIFFERENTIAL DIAGNOSIS:

If the test result is HIGH:

> phenylalanine metabolism in the body is blocked,
> causing phenylketonuria (PKU) and possible
> mental retardation; false-positive because of use of
> antibiotic (ampicillin).

If the test result is LOW:

> no evidence of phenylalanine metabolism abnormality.

COMMENT: PKU (phenylketonuria) testing is done
routinely on every baby born in a hospital in the
United States by law. The test is done from a drop of
blood absorbed onto a piece of filter paper shortly

after birth and the infant has started feeding (48-72 hours after birth). The test is very sensitive and specific, and is done because the PKU test identifies babies who have a genetic abnormality that has to do with the metabolism of an important amino acid, phenylalanine. If the phenylalanine level is too high, mental retardation occurs in a high percentage of the babies so affected. However, it is important to understand that not *all* individuals with elevated phenylalanine in the blood have phenylketonuria.

Unfortunately, not all babies are born in a hospital where the test is performed. Therefore those infants and children who have not been tested should be tested for PKU as soon as possible well before the age of ten years during the period of brain development, and obviously the sooner the better. When this disease is uncovered by testing, lifelong dietary management can be started that will control the level of phenylalanine in the body.

Pregnant women who are genetic carriers of the disease must be tested for PKU, because high levels of phenylalanine in the mother can result in mental retardation in her baby. If there is no record of PKU testing (e.g., a foreign born woman who was born in a hospital that did not test for PKU, or where hospital records were poorly kept), the test should be performed early in pregnancy.

FOLLOW-UP: If PKU has not been done for some reason, it should be done at the first visit to a well-baby clinic or visit to a physician. Dietary therapy is the only presently effective management plan. This should be carried out under medical supervision with nutritionist consultation where this is possible.

Parents names should be entered into the database of a genetic register for the disease.

3. RANDOM BLOOD GLUCOSE (SUGAR)

TYPICAL WORRY: *There's a history of diabetes in the family, and I want to make sure my twelve year old son hasn't inherited it.*

TEST: Random Blood Glucose (Sugar)

TEST RESULTS: (*example*) 256 mg/dL (SI: 8.7 mmol/L)

URGENCY LEVEL: Action: √ Decision:

NORMAL RANGE: 2 years to Adult: < 200 mg/dL (SI: <11.1 mmol/L)

ORIGIN OR SOURCE OF SUBSTANCES TESTED FOR: glucose (sugar) in a blood or plasma sample.

DIFFERENTIAL DIAGNOSIS:

If test results are HIGH, >200 mg/dL (SI: >11.1 mmol/L) or higher:

> impairment of glucose tolerance as a result of:
> diabetes mellitus
> non-fasting blood specimen

If test results are LOW, < 50 mg/dL (SI: < 2.8 mmol/L):

a diabetic who has injected too much insulin
> pancreatic or other tumors
> liver disease
> malnutrition (e.g., anorexia nervosa) or starvation
> hormonal disorder related to the adrenal or pituitary
> gland.

COMMENT: *Glucose* is synonymous with *sugar* in the blood. Because it is often inconvenient or difficult to have a blood sugar test done after the necessary eight hours of fasting required for a Fasting Blood Sugar (FBS), most blood sugar tests are done *randomly* and are referred to as *Random Blood Sugar. Fasting Blood* Sugar test values are usually quite different from Random Blood Sugar test results.

Any HIGH blood sugar results should be retested after fasting for eight hours, or done as a 2 hour *postprandial* (after eating) Blood Glucose test, or by a Glucose Tolerance Test (*see Chapter 15, GTT*).

A high-risk child or adolescent—overweight, or who has a close relative with diabetes—should have Random Blood Glucose tests annually. Children who are proven to be diabetics—usually Type I, insulin dependent ("IDDM")—should have their treatment program carefully followed, and in addition to Random Blood Glucose tests, a Hemoglobin A1c test should be done every three months (*see Chapter 15, Hemoglobin A1c*) which will indicate how well blood glucose levels have been controlled in the previous three months.

FOLLOW-UP: Call or see your doctor if your child's test result is out of the normal range. Your physician may choose to do additional tests to rule out causes other than diabetes in the above Differential Diagnoses for the abnormal blood sugar test result. If his or her Hemoglobin A1c test result is higher than 6%, the child's blood sugar level has not been optimally controlled and must be taken by the child's physician to bring the blood sugar to appropriate levels to prevent or forestall development of the serious complications of this disease.

4. SEXUALLY TRANSMITTED DISEASE (STD)

TYPICAL WORRY: *I know my 15 year old daughter is sexually active and now she has a discharge. I'm scared that she may have some awful disease she got from sex.*

Adolescents and young adults may be victims of a moral code that prevails in much of the world which is increasingly tolerant of sexual freedom without insistence on responsibility for that freedom. The unfortunate result is unexpected and unwanted pregnancies, and the spread of Sexually Transmitted Disease (STD). Many of these diseases have serious and often permanent consequences for those so engaged; examples are HIV infection, AIDS, gonorrhea, (often causing infertility due to scarring of fallopian tubes), chlamydia, and other chronic illnesses previously referred to as venereal disease (VD).

Too few STD-infected adolescents are treated for these diseases before it is too late because of the embarrassment and fear of the afflicted about revealing their sexual activities to parents, counselors, friends, and physicians. Parents must have a high index of suspicion concerning an adolescent's behavior, friends, and social activities. The "ostrich" approach, assuming or hoping that "my child would never be engaged in anything like that" is a popular but very naive belief.

The reality is that Nature imprints all humans with the requirements for species survival, exhibited by the surge of powerful hormones at the onset of puberty. The desire for sexual activity is real—and normal. Understanding and recognizing this reality is essential to influencing behavior. Eternal vigilance, communication, and openness to the adolescents *of both sexes* about sexual matters and prevention of an unwanted pregnancy is a parental responsibility and challenge.

Listed in Chapter 23 are the readily available laboratory tests that can be used to identify STD in individuals at all ages. Be aware that your adolescent may already be using these laboratory services through a walk-in, perhaps store-front office run by Planned Parenthood or other organizations concerned with the realities of teen-age behavior. Such facilities often are low profile in a community, and are frequently staffed by nurse practitioners trained in the handling of adolescents with a problem of pregnancy, contraception, STD, or the need for counseling in how to deal with someone of the opposite sex who wants to engage in sexual activity.

Please refer to Chapter 23, Sexually Transmitted Disease for the list of tests that may be used in diagnosing the presence of these diseases.

5. TOTAL CHOLESTEROL (TC)

TYPICAL WORRY: *I wonder if my son's cholesterol is high. I'm concerned because both my father and my brother have had heart attacks and have high cholesterol.*

TEST: Blood cholesterol and cholesterol fractions

TEST RESULTS: (example is for a 10 year old boy)
Total cholesterol (TC): 225 mg/dL (SI: 5.8 mmol/L)
Cholesterol fractions:
HDLC ("good") cholesterol: 23 mg/dL (SI: 0.6 mmol/L)
LDLC ("bad") cholesterol: 133 mg/dL (SI: 3.4 mmol/L)
TC:HDL ratio: 9.78
LDLC:HDLC: 5.78

URGENCY LEVEL: Action: __√__ Decision: _____

AVERAGE VALUES:

Age-related Average Values for Total Cholesterol

Age:	0-19	20-29	30-39	>39
TC mg/dL:	155 (4.0)	175 (4.5)	195 (5.1)	210 (5.4)
(approximate HDLC mg/dL:	50 (1.3)	45 (1.2)	45 (1.2)	50 (1.3)
mean values) LDLC mg/dL:	95 (2.5)	110 (3.2)	130 (3.4)	145 (3.9)

ORIGIN OR SOURCE OF SUBSTANCES TESTED FOR: substances produced by cells in the body; influenced by genetics, diet, exercise, chronic alcohol ingestion, hormones, or medications.

DIFFERENTIAL DIAGNOSIS:

If the test results are HIGH:

> primary hyperlipoproteinemia (genetic predisposition); secondary hyperlipoproteinemia due to kidney disease; hypothyroidism; diabetes; obesity; lack of exercise; use of drugs such as steroids, beta blockers, thiazides.

If the test results are LOW:

> severe liver disease; malabsorption of dietary nutrients; malnutrition; hyperthryroidism.

COMMENT: All persons under age 20 should have their Total Cholesterol tested at least once as a screening test to detect a possible genetic predisposition to coronary artery disease, and thereafter tested every five years. Those found to have abnormally high cholesterol should have a Cardiac Risk Analysis (*see Chapter 16, Heart Disease Tests*) performed to find abnormalities early enough so that protective measures can be taken to prevent the development of coronary artery or other vascular disease.

Table 8 indicates "average American" risk.

Table 8

Cardiac Risk Based on TC:HDLC Ratio

Risk Level	Male	Female
1/2 average	3.4-4.9	3.3-4.3
average	5.0-9.5	4.4-6.9
2 X average	9.6-23.3	7.0-10.9
3 X average	> 23.3	> 10.9

Average values for Americans are higher than average values for many other geographically or ethnically distinct groups of people worldwide. American average Total Cholesterol values would be considered abnormally high to physicians in many other parts of the world.

Only one or two test results may be abnormal while others are within normal range. Concentrate on improving any abnormal values so that all test results are within normal range.

It is now clear that "statins" are very helpful in lowering high cholesterol, especially when combined with appropriate life style behavior.

Cholesterol elevation in children and adolescents is often controllable by diet, exercise, and establishing lifetime good lifestyle habits. If drug therapy (e.g., "statins") is necessary, it should be under medical supervision.

FOLLOW-UP: Call or see your doctor for advice if your child's test results are outside normal ranges. Be sure to discuss any abnormalities and their possible relationship to medications your child may be taking, and make your child aware of the significance of these test results.

CHAPTER 18

Legal-Issue Tests

1. Blood Alcohol

2. Paternity Test Panel

3. Prostatic Acid Phosphatase (PAP)

1. BLOOD ALCOHOL

TYPICAL WORRY: *I flunked the breath test the State Trooper gave me, but I only had one or two beers. I want a blood test.*

TEST: Alcohol (ethanol) in Blood (Blood Alchohol)

TEST RESULTS: (*example*) 50mg/dL (SI:10.9mmol/L).

URGENCY LEVEL: Action: __√__ Decision: _____

NORMAL RANGE: Blood:<10mg/dL) (SI: <10.9mmol/L).

ORIGIN OR SOURCE OF SUBSTANCE TESTED FOR: alcohol (ethanol) ingested recreationally.

DIFFERENTIAL DIAGNOSIS:

If test results are HIGH:

Diseases: acute and/or chronic alcoholism
Legal problem: Driving While Intoxicated (DWI)

If test results are 0.0, "NEGATIVE", OR "WITHIN LEGAL LIMIT":

you are *not* legally intoxicated.

COMMENT: Standards for determining intoxication by alcohol vary from state to state; whether you were DWI or not legally depends upon the established statutory definition for alcoholic intoxication in the state or locality where the presumed offense was committed. Most clinical laboratories report alcohol in mg/dL, but many state laws classify the degree of intoxication by *percent of weight/volume*, this can be confusing. In many states, anything at or above 0.10% (equivalent to 10mg/dL) is considered to be evidence of some degree of alcoholic intoxiation. It is assumed that in many individuals alcohol in the blood at this level implies impaired judgment, slowed reaction time, and loss of inhibitions to some degree. Urine alcohol content is less useful information and probably would not be helpful in court.

Be sure to get copies of any test reports or data the police have obtained (e.g., breath, blood, or alcohol test results, etc.); you are entitled to these.

If you are an alcoholic and are concerned about liver disease, liver function tests are available (*see Chapter 11, Liver Panel*).

FOLLOW-UP: Whether or not your blood alchohol test result is abnormal, *call your attorney at once* if you think you may need to produce this information in a court of law. An attorney can advise you on how to proceed to handle this embarrassment. Even if you are sober now, but you are an alcoholic, be sure to let your healthcare provider know. He or she can help you get treatment for this serious health problem—and perhaps that will help you get your license to drive restored!

2. PATERNITY TEST PANEL

TYPICAL WORRY: *I know I'm not the father of my ex-girl friend's baby.*

TESTS: Human leukocyte antigens (HLA) typing; Identification desoxyribonucleic acid (DNA) testing; Blood grouping and typing (ABO and Rh).

TEST RESULTS: (*example*) HLA typing: parentage excluded. Identification DNA Testing: parentage excluded (99.99% probability); ABO and Rh: parentage excluded.

URGENCY LEVEL: Action: __√__ Decision: _____

NORMAL RANGE: (Not applicable)

ORIGIN OR SOURCE OF SUBSTANCES TEST FOR:

> HLA: human white blood cells;
> DNA: whole blood, amniotic fluid, tissue; semen;
> ABO—Rh: whole blood.

DIFFERENTIAL DIAGNOSIS:

> If "parentage excluded": individual is not one of the parents.
> If "parentage can be neither excluded nor proven": individual could or could not be one of the parents.
> If "possibility of parentage cannot be excluded entirely": probability of parentage is highly unlikely.

COMMENT: Folks who study these things have declared that perhaps ten percent of the population in the United

States is mistaken concerning who their father really is. Thus it is not surprising that the question comes up fairly frequently, and the question can only be resolved with certainty by the use of laboratory tests and legal counsel. The lawyers love it.

In cases of rape, there are two questions at issue: the first is whether there is evidence of the presence or absence of semen in the raped person's genitalia or clothing; this may often be resolved by using the relatively inexpensive Prostatic Acid Phosphatase test (PAP) (*see following in this Chapter*). The second question is, whose semen is it? Here is where DNA testing is of great value in resolving the problem of identity. This task is best performed in accredited forensic (legal) medical laboratories specializing in this type of testing.

Testing (except for ABO and Rh blood grouping) can be expensive. It is reasonable to have the court decide who is to pay for the laboratory tests used in paternity testing—accused or accuser, winner or loser—or whether there is to be a sharing. DNA testing is very expensive, but it is presently the "gold standard" for establishing identity.

The tests used for parentage testing can also be applied to other questions of parentage (e.g., hospital nursery mix-ups, kidnaps, etc.). In any event, maintenance of a *documented chain of custody* of specimens throughout the collection, transport, test performance, as well as the recording of test results within the laboratory sequence is essential if test results are to be admissible as evidence in a court of law.

FOLLOW-UP: An attorney's advice is strongly urged upon anyone wishing to resolve a question relating to parentage.

3. PROSTATIC ACID PHOSPHATASE (PAP)

TYPICAL WORRY: *I have been acused of rape. It is not true!*

TESTS: Prostatic acid phosphatase (PAP)

TEST RESULT: (*example*) 23.0 U/L (SI: same)

URGENCY LEVEL: Action: _√_ Decision: _____

NORMAL RANGE: (forensic: 0.0)

ORIGIN OR SOURCE OF SUBSTANCES TEST FOR: an enzyme produced by cells in the prostate gland and present in male semen

DIFFERENTIAL DIAGNOSIS:

If test results are POSITIVE at any concentration:

> presumptive evidence of the presence of semen.

If test result is NEGATIVE:

> no evidence of semen.

COMMENT: PAP in vaginal secretions(or on clothing) is tested for in cases of alleged rape; the presence of PAP in vaginal secretions is presumptive evidence that genital penetration and ejaculation of semen have occured, but its absence does not prove that rape has not occured—a condom could have been used by an assailant. Also, PAP does not identify the individual who may have been the source of the semen. This would require DNA testing (*see Paternity Test Panel, foregoing in this Chapter*).

As with any forensic investigations, maintenance of a *documented chain of custody* of specimens throughout the collection, transport, test performance, as well as the recording of test results within the laboratory sequence is essential if test results are to be admissible as evidence in a court of law.

FOLLOW-UP: Any allegation of rape is obviously a serious matter, and the sooner legal assistance is obtained the better. Rape is an accusation with dire consequences for the person if he is proven beyond reasonable doubt to have committed the crime. Therefore an accused male's attorney might decide to have the PAP as well as any DNA testing repeated at another laboratory of the accused's choice to verify all test results.

CHAPTER 19

Libido Test

1. Total Testosterone

1. TOTAL TESTOSTERONE

TYPICAL WORRY: *My interest in sex has just about disappeared and my husband is very unhappy about that. Many of my friends who are past the menopause say that they haven't had this problem.*

TEST: Total testosterone

TEST RESULT: (*examples*)

> Total testosterone:
> *female*: 10 ng/dL (SI: 0.4 nmol/L)

URGENCY LEVEL: Action: __√__ Decision: _____

NORMAL RANGES:

> Total testosterone:
> *female*: 20-80 ng/dL (SI: 0.7-2.8 nmol/L)
> *male*: 300-1200 ng/dL (SI: 10.4-41.6 nmol/L)
> 200-300 ng/dL, (SI: 6.9-10.4 nmol/L) borderline
> low < 200 ng/dL (SI: < 6.9 nmol/L), deficient level.

ORIGIN OR SOURCE OF SUBSTANCES TESTED FOR: a hormone produced predominantly by the male testes (testicles) and in much smaller amount by the adrenal glands and ovaries in females.

DIFFERENTIAL DIAGNOSIS:

If *female* total testosterone is HIGH:

> polycystic ovary syndrome; if very HIGH (> 200 ng/dL, SI: 70 nmol/L), tumor of ovary or adrenal gland.

If *female* total testosterone level is LOW:

> menopause, with or without decreased libido (sex drive).

If *male* total testosterone is LOW:

> erectile dysfunction (ED) (can't get or maintain a penile erection); illness such as diabetes, AIDS, some testicular cancers; medication for treatment of prostate gland cancer; natural progression of decline in hormone level due to aging.

COMMENT: There is a balancing of sex hormone levels during life that relates to "maleness", "femaleness", and libido. Recent studies suggest that loss of libido, especially in older women, but also in some men, may be associated with abnormally low testosterone levels that might be responsive to hormonal therapy.

Some male physicians do not feel comfortable discussing matters like libido with their female patients so they do not ask questions about it. Unfortunately, many, perhaps most, older women are embarrassed to bring the subject up with a male doctor who is neither a gynecologist nor a psychiatrist because of the cultural bias in our society against discussing sexuality or related matters openly, even with a physician. Female nurse practitioners are perhaps more likely to discuss matters related to sexual activity with women.

There is still insufficient information about the use of testosterone (or Viagra™, which is *not* testosterone) therapy for loss of libido in women or men, especially older men, to state whether or not the advantages outweigh the liabilities. Most physicians feel that more research is needed. It is generally accepted that testosterone therapy for men may be indicated only when a man with ED has a normal prostate gland by digital rectal examination (DRE) and a normal PSA test level (*see Chapter 22, Prostate Specific Antigen*).

FOLLOW-UP: Call or see your doctor, who may order other tests to establish a diagnosis, and who can decide whether or not you should be on the hormone replacement therapy (HRT)—if any—appropriate for you. Do not be afraid to discuss your sexuality worries and concerns with your healthcare provider. If you don't get help, find someone who will discuss these concerns with you. Women physicians and female nurse practitioners are often more approachable on these subjects than male physicians.

CHAPTER 20

Menopause Tests

1. Menopause Panel
   Estrogens
   Luteinizing Hormones
   Papanicalou Smear Maturation
   Index

1. MENOPAUSE PANEL

TYPICAL WORRY: *I think I'm going into the menopause, but I'm not sure if I should be on hormone replacement therapy. My periods are very irregular, and my interest in sex has disappeared.*

TESTS: Urinary Estrogens (E1-estrone; E2-estradiol; E3-estriol; E4-estrol); the test includes urine volume and creatinine concentration in urine; Luteinizing Hormone (LH); Papanicalou Smear Maturation Index (MI).

TEST RESULTS: (*examples*)

> Estrogens: 12 µg/24 hrs (SI: 42 µmol/day);
> Luteinizing Hormone: 4 mIU/mL (SI: 4 IU/L);
> Pap Smear Maturation Index: 60/30/10.

URGENCY LEVEL: Action: __√__ Decision: _____

NORMAL RANGE:

> Estrogens (from 24 hour urine sample):
> *menstruating:* 15-18 µg/24 hrs (SI: 52-277 µmol/day);
> *menopause:* < 20 µg/24 hrs (SI: < 69 µmol/day);
> Luteinizing Hormone: 6-30 mIU/mL (SI: 6-30 IU/L)
> Pap Smear Maturation Index: varies with menstrual
>   cycle in ovulating women (percentages are
>   approximate):
> 0/40/60: *preovulatory;*
> 0/70/30: *premenstrual;*
> 65/30/5: early menopause (~ age 45-60):
> 100/0/0: late menopause (~ age 60 and older).

ORIGIN OR SOURCE OF SUBSTANCES TESTED FOR:
Estrogens are produced by ovaries; Luteinizing
Hormone is produced by the pituitary gland; Pap
Smear: cells shed from the surface of the vagina and
cervix.

DIFFERENTIAL DIAGNOSIS:

If Estrogens and Luteinizing Hormone are HIGH:

certain tumors of the ovary;

If Luteinizing Hormone alone is HIGH:

ovarian failure; menopause; following oophorectomy
(surgical ovary removal).

If Estrogen test result is LOW:

ovarian failure to produce hormones (various
causes); infertility; premenopause; menopause;
menstrual irregularities.

COMMENT: Decreased ovarian hormonal production usually
comes on gradually. Occasionally there is a precipitous
drop in female hormones and menopause ceases
abruptly, but this is the exception rather than the
rule. Many factors and complex hormone interactions
make specific diagnoses based on hormonal assays
difficult, and often only by evaluating trends in test
results can a physician reach a conclusion concerning
diagnosis. Decreased libido does not correlate closely
with the onset of menopause and is more closely
correlated with levels of total testosterone (*see Chapter
19, Libido*).

A relatively inexpensive way to assess hormonal function is through the Maturation Index portion of a Pap Smear report. The cells lining the female genital tract change their appearance in response to hormonal stimulation (or the lack of it), and the relative percentages of cells in various stages of maturation can be used as an index of hormone production. If an MI is not routinely included in your Pap Smear report, you or your doctor can request that this be done on previous and future smears.

Hormone tests usually require the collection of all urine produced over a 24 hour period. An appropriate container and instructions about collecting the urine are supplied by the clinical laboratory performing the test.

FOLLOW-UP: Whether or not you should be receiving HRT that is appropriate for your hormonal status must be decided by you with the help of your doctor. Hot flashes and other unpleasant aspects of menopause can usually be controlled medically, but it is important that the risks associated with certain hormones or combinations of hormones be known, understood, and accepted before a treatment program is started.

CHAPTER 21

Pregnancy and Infertility Tests

1. Alpha1-fetoprotein

2. Cystic Fibrosis Screening:
   Chloride Sweat Test

3. Folic Acid (Folate)

4. Human Chorionic
   Gonadotropin (hCG)

5. Pregnancy Test on Urine

6. Prenatal Test Panel
   ABO and Rh typing
   Antiglobulin Test
   Folic Acid (Folate)

7. Progesterone

8. Semen Analysis for Infertility
   or Post-vasectomy Check

1. ALPHA1-FETOPROTEIN

TYPICAL WORRY: *I'm a 42 year old pregnant woman, and I want to make sure my baby is going to be normal and not have one of those awful genetic diseases.*

TEST: Alpha1-fetoprotein.

TEST RESULTS: (*example*) 3 ng/mL (SI: 3 µg/L)

URGENCY LEVEL: Action: __√__ Decision: _____

NORMAL RANGE: depends on mother's race, body weight, and length of pregnancy.

ORIGIN OR SOURCE OF SUBSTANCES TESTED FOR: a protein present in the fetal (baby's) blood, and transported through the placenta to maternal (mother's) blood.

DIFFERENTIAL DIAGNOSIS:

If the test result is HIGH:

> possible abnormalities in the fetus (e.g., spina bifida, neural tube—the part of the developing fetus that gives rise to the brain and spinal cord—defects, absence of fetal head or brain; dead fetus); pre-eclampsia (a serious toxic condition of the mother occurring late in pregnancy).

If the test result is LOW:

> possible Down syndrome.

COMMENT: The mother's blood for this test *must* be collected between the 16th and 18th week of pregnancy. Only a physician experienced in obstetrical patient management should interpret the rather complicated laboratory report for this test.

This is an important screening test that can be done on either maternal blood or amniotic fluid ("bag of waters" surrounding the fetus in the uterus). The test is especially important for older women who are pregnant, since fetal abnormalities are more likely to occur in women in the 30-45+ year age range.

FOLLOW-UP: Older women who are pregnant should be carefully supervised during pregnancy, since complications of pregnancy and abnormalities of the fetus occur more frequently than in younger pregnant women. Ultrasound studies of the fetus and examination of the amniotic fluid after amniocentesis (the insertion of a needle into the bag of waters surrounding the baby to obtain amniotic fluid for genetic examination) provide useful information about the baby, including its sex; these studies may be suggested or ordered by the physician.

2. CHLORIDE SWEAT TEST

TYPICAL WORRY: *I'm pregnant and there is cystic fibrosis in my family. I don't want to have a baby with that disease.*

TEST: Chloride Sweat Test.

TEST RESULTS: (*example*) 65 mmol/L. (SI: 65 mmol/L).

URGENCY LEVEL: Action: __√__ Decision: _____

NORMAL RANGE: 0-40 mmol/L (SI: 0-40 mmol/L).

ORIGIN OR SOURCE OF SUBSTANCE TESTED FOR: chloride in the sweat excreted through the skin after application of a medication on the skin.

DIFFERENTIAL DIAGNOSIS:

If the test results are HIGH:

> age 0-20 yrs.: > 60 mmol/L (SI: same)
> age 20+: > 70 mmol/L (SI: same), then cystic fibrosis (CF) must be seriously considered, especially if CF symptoms exist.

If test results are LOW:

> cystic fibrosis cannot be excluded with certainty, but is unlikely.

COMMENT: This relatively inexpensive test is an aid in diagnosing CF, and is not a definitive test. Cystic fibrosis is likely if high Sweat Chloride is associated with foul-smelling stools, frequent bouts of pneumonia, chronic cough, (and in infants and children: failure-to-thrive, asthma, and frequent or severe gastrointestinal problems). Screening for the disease in a pregnant woman who does not have symptoms of CF may not exclude the possibility of her baby having CF if she or the father are carriers of CF genes. The Cystic Fibrosis DNA Content test is more definitive than the Chloride Sweat Test if CF is suspected because of signs and symptoms of the disease (*see Chapter 15, Cystic Fibrosis DNA Content*).

FOLLOW-UP: Call your doctor. Your physician will choose the tests, if any, that may be necessary as an aid in the diagnosis of latent or overt CF. The Cystic Fibrosis DNA Content test is often recommended for pregnant women to determine whether or not they are genetic carriers for the disease. If both parents are carriers, the probability of CF in the child is higher than if neither, or only one, parent is a carrier.

3. FOLIC ACID (FOLATE)

TYPICAL WORRY: *I want to get pregnant, and I've heard from my sister that my baby may have birth defects if I don't have enough folic acid in my body early in pregnancy.*

TEST: Folic acid (folate)

TEST RESULTS: (*example*) 0.7 ng/mL (SI: 1.6nmol/L)

URGENCY LEVEL: Action: __√__ Decision: _____

NORMAL RANGE: > 2 ng/mL (SI: > 4.5 nmol/L)

ORIGIN OR SOURCE OF SUBSTANCES TESTED FOR: a B-complex vitamin present in a wide variety of foods and included in most OTC multivitamin pills.

DIFFERENTIAL DIAGNOSIS:

If the test result is HIGH:

of little clinical significance.

If the test result is LOW:

low dietary intake; megaloblastic (pernicious) anemia; chronic alcoholism; Crohn's disease; intestinal malabsorption syndrome.

COMMENT: Unsuspected folic acid deficiency is common in pregnancy (said to be about 33%) and can be associated with serious adverse effects on the fetus. Pregnant women or those contemplating pregnancy should take folic acid supplement, especially before and during the first trimester (0-14 weeks) of pregnancy. (Pernicious anemia can be diagnosed only when the folic acid test result fits in with other clinical abnormalities; the folic acid test result alone is not specifically diagnostic of pernicious anemia).

FOLLOW-UP: Call or see your doctor for advice about prenatal care if you are pregnant.

4. SERUM HUMAN CHORIONIC GONADOTROPIN (ßHCG)

TYPICAL WORRY: *I've missed my menstrual period, and I don't know whether I'm starting menopause or I'm pregnant again.*

TEST: Beta (β) subunit Human Chorionic Gonadotropin.

TEST RESULT: (*example*) 6.5 mIU/ml (SI: 6.5 IU/L).

URGENCY LEVEL: Action: __√__ Decision: _____

NORMAL RANGE: Negative, or < 3 mIU/mL (SI: < 3 IU/L).

ORIGIN OR SOURCE OF SUBSTANCE TESTED FOR: a substance (glycoprotein) secreted by the cells forming the fetus's (baby's) placenta and present in the mother's blood and urine.

DIFFERENTIAL DIAGNOSIS:

If the test results are HIGH (exceed 3 mIU/mL):

0-14 weeks gestation (pregnancy)—viable (normal) pregnancy.

If test results are LOW or HAVE FALLEN:

abortion* ("miscarriage"); threatened abortion (possibility of miscarriage); ectopic pregnancy (i.e., outside the uterus, usually in a fallopian tube, referred to then as a "tubal pregnancy").

COMMENT: Most medical laboratories offer a *quantitative* blood serum test that measures the amount of hCG and gives test results in International Units (IU). Pregnancy is diagnosed as pregnant when the test result exceeds 3 IU/L. hCG levels.

Over the counter (OTC) pregnancy test kits on urine are usually *qualitative*—they give a Positive or Negative test result, and are not useful in monitoring the progression of a pregnancy.

Serial quantitative tests on blood or urine are useful in determining trends in hCG levels, which normally increase rapidly during the first trimester (14 weeks) of pregnancy. A leveling off or fall in hCG test results suggests that a presumed normal pregnancy is not going well and that miscarriage will possibly occur.

FOLLOW-UP: If test results are POSITIVE or there are signs of pregnancy, early prenatal care is essential to the well-being of both mother and fetus. If there are symptoms or signs of abnormality early or late in pregnancy (e.g., cramps, vaginal spotting or bleeding), a physician should be seen at once. He or she may order hCG levels and/or other tests in order to plan proper management of the pregnancy.

* "abortion" is the *medical* term for the termination of a pregnancy by either natural or induced means; "abortion" as used *politically* and in the media usually means a pregnancy purposely ended by choice; this would be referred to *medically* as an "induced abortion".

5. PREGNANCY TESTS

TYPICAL WORRY: *I've missed my period and I think I'm pregnant.*

TEST: Urinary beta human chorionic gonadotropin (βhCG)

TEST RESULTS: (*example*) Positive

URGENCY LEVEL: Action: __√__ Decision: _____

NORMAL RANGE: Negative: not pregnant

ORIGIN OR SOURCE OF SUBSTANCE TESTED FOR: a
    substance secreted by the cells forming the fetus's
    (baby's) placenta and present in the mother's blood
    and urine.

DIFFERENTIAL DIAGNOSIS:

If the test is NEGATIVE:

    not pregnant

If test results are POSITIVE:

    pregnant

COMMENT: Urine test kits can be bought over-the-counter
    (OTC) without a prescription or doctor's order.
    These are *qualitative* tests that test for the presence
    or absence of βhCG. The pregnancy test most often
    done in medical laboratories is a *quantitative* test that
    measures the amount of bhCG present in blood
    serum (*see in this Chapter*) and serves a different
    purpose than the "yes-or-no" OTC qualitative urine

test. Presently available OTC test kits are quite sensitive and reliable—but not fool-proof. Many years ago this test was a biological test using live frogs or rabbits, and was then known as the "frog test" or "rabbit test"; these were far less reliable than today's chemical test.

Pregnancy tests are important screening tests to be certain that a patient is not pregnant who is about to have surgery or in whom radioactive or chemotherapeutic agents ("chemo") are to be used.

FOLLOW-UP: If pregnancy is shown by testing, prenatal care by a physician or midwife is essential to assure a safe and successful outcome. Special test or studies (e.g., serum bhCG, serum progesterone, ultrasound, amniocentesis, folic acid) may be ordered if a physician suspects a complication in the pregnancy.

If there are symptoms or signs of abnormality early or late in pregnancy (e.g., cramps, vaginal spotting or bleeding), a physician should be seen at once. He or she may order serum bhCG levels and/or other tests in order to plan proper management of the pregnancy.

6. PRENATAL TEST PANEL

TYPICAL WORRY: *I'm pregnant again, and I know I should get some lab tests done. My husband and I are of different blood types.*

TEST PANEL: Blood ABO and Rh_0 (D) grouping (typing)
Folic acid (Folate)
Antiglobulin test ("Coombs test").

TEST RESULTS: (*example*) Blood group (type): AB, Rh_0- ("AB, Negative") Folic Acid: 7.0 ng/mL (SI: 17.6 nmol/L) Antiglobulin test: Positive

URGENCY LEVEL: Action: √ Decision:

NORMAL RANGE: (not applicable for blood grouping)
Folic acid: > 2.7 ng/mL (SI: > 6.8 nmol/L)
Antiglobulin test: Negative

ORIGIN OR SOURCE OF SUBSTANCE TESTED FOR: *Blood groups*: specific substances (antigens) present on all red blood cells (RBC); *folic acid*: a B-complex vitamin; *antiglobulin*: an antibody that combines with and precipitates the protein globulin.

DIFFERENTIAL DIAGNOSIS:

Blood grouping:

If a woman tests Rh_0 (D) POSITIVE:

> *not* susceptible to sensitization by the Rh_0 (D) antigen, and her baby will *not* develop *hemolytic disease of the newborn* (HDN) due to Rh incompatibility.

If a woman tests Rh_0 (D) NEGATIVE:

> she *is* susceptible to sensitization by the Rh_0 (D) antigen, and her baby *could* develop *hemolytic disease of the newborn* (HDN) due to Rh incompatibility.

Folic acid:

If folic acid is HIGH:

> adequate amount of the vitamin in the body;

If folic acid is LOW:

> deficient amount of the vitamin in the body with possible adverse effects on the fetus such as mental retardation.

Antiglobulin test:

If the test is NEGATIVE:

> *sensitization* has not taken place and HDN due to Rh_0 incompatibility is unlikely;

If the test is POSITIVE:

> the mother is *sensitized,* with possible destruction of the fetus's red blood cells; HDN is a possible serious consequence.

COMMENT: If a woman tests $Rh_0(D)$ *negative* (and/or *Du negative*) and her baby is $Rh_0(D)$ *positive,* she is susceptible to possible *sensitization* (similar to developing an allergy) because of the incompatibility of her blood Rh group and the blood Rh group of her baby (i.e., mother is "Rh negative" and her baby is "Rh positive"). As a result of this incompatibility the baby may be born with *hemolytic disease of the newborn* (HDN), (also called *erythroblastosis fetalis*). HDN is a serious disease in which there is destruction of the baby's red blood cells while in the uterus and after birth that could result in illness or death of the newborn if undetected early and untreated, *It can be prevented during proper early prenatal care!*

While less common and usually less serious, ABO sensitization can occur, because of ABO maternal-fetal blood group incompatibility (e.g., mother is group A, baby is group B), *regardless* of whether she is Rh_0 negative or Rh_0 positive. It is recommended that ABO and Rh type be tested for *early in pregnancy*, and that an antiglobulin test ("Coombs" test) be done in early *and* late pregnancy in all women who are $RH_0(D)$ negative and have not been previously immunized with *Rh immune globulin* as part of their prenatal care.

FOLLOW-UP: Early prenatal care is essential to the well-being of both mother and fetus. If there are symptoms or signs of abnormality early or late in pregnancy (e.g., cramps, vaginal spotting or bleeding), a physician should be seen at once. He or she may order βhCG and progesterone levels and/or other tests in order to plan proper management of the pregnancy.

It is *important* that an antiglobulin test be done after miscarriage of an Rh_0 negative woman, to check for evidence of possible sensitization of the mother by the aborted fetus.

7. PROGESTERONE

TYPICAL WORRY: *I'm pregnant again after losing my three previous pregnancies. I'm worried that I might lose this one too.*

TEST: Progesterone

TEST RESULT: (*example*) 25 ng/mL (SI: 79.5 nmol/L)

URGENCY LEVEL: Action: __√__ Decision: _____

SIGNIFICANT RANGES:

> normal pregnancy: = or > 25 ng/mL (SI: = or > 79.5 nmol/L)
> abnormal pregnancy: < 10 ng/mL (SI: < 31.8 nmol/L)
> non-viable (dead) fetus: < 5 ng/mL (SI: < 15.9 nmol/L)

ORIGIN OR SOURCE OF SUBSTANCES TESTED FOR: a hormone secreted by the ovary and by the placenta after pregnancy is established.

DIFFERENTIAL DIAGNOSIS:

If the test result is HIGH (= or > 20 ng/mL, SI: > 63.6 nmol/L) during the first trimester (0-14 weeks) and continues to rise on subsequent testing:

> outlook for a successful pregnancy is favorable.

If the test result is LOW (< 20 ng/mL, SI: < 63.6 nmol/L) during the first trimester (0-14 weeks) and fails to rise or falls on subsequent testing:

pregnancy in jeopardy; ectopic (outside the uterus) pregnancy.

COMMENT: Progesterone is essential to the maintenance and progression of a normal pregnancy. Failure of the ovary to produce progesterone in adequate amount may influence ovulation (the release of an egg from the ovary) and be a cause of infertility and habitual abortion. Progesterone is a useful test in monitoring pregnancy, but the test may not be available from all laboratories.

FOLLOW-UP: Call or see your doctor for advice about prenatal care if you are pregnant; call at once if you suspect miscarriage because of cramps, or vaginal spotting or bleeding.

8. SEMEN ANALYSIS

TYPICAL WORRY: *My wife and I have been trying to have a family without any luck. Her gynecologist suggested that I have a fertility test.*

TEST: Semen analysis.

TEST RESULTS: (*example*)

Volume:	3.0 mL
Color:	grey-white
Clotting and Liquefaction:	35 minutes
pH:	7.2
Sperm count:	29 million/mL
Sperm motility:	45%
Sperm morphology:	44 % normal forms

URGENCY LEVEL: Action: _√_ Decision: _____

NORMAL RANGES:

Volume:	2-5 mL
Color:	grey-white or white
Clotting and Liquefaction:	complete in 30 minutes
pH:	7.1-7.2
Sperm count:	50-150 million/mL
Sperm motility:	60%
Sperm morphology:	= or > 70% normal forms

ORIGIN OR SOURCE OF SUBSTANCES TESTED FOR: sperm (spermatocytes) produced in the testes; secretions from the prostate and urethral glands.

DIFFERENTIAL DIAGNOSIS:

If the Sperm count is HIGH:

> no significance.

If the Sperm count is LOW, or morphology includes TOO FEW NORMAL FORMS, or the motility is LOW:

> infertility of the male may be suspected.

COMMENT: *Infertility Testing*: Abnormalities of sperm production in the testes (testicles, balls) may be the consequence of illnesses in childhood (e.g., mumps, or high fevers) that have caused testicular damage or atrophy. Semen abnormalities may also be due to the use of street drugs (e.g., marijuana, cocaine, crack, etc.). Abnormalities in volume, pH, clotting, etc. may relate to alterations in secretions of the prostate gland; causes for such changes are not well understood, but may relate to body chemistry (e.g., diabetes), or reflect hormonal insufficiencies or imbalances.

> *Post-Vasectomy Check*: If the Semen Analysis is to assure that a vasectomy operation was successful in eliminating sperm from the semen, the Sperm Count test result should be "Zero" or "0". If sperm are present, the surgeon performing the surgery should be informed immediately; he or she will undoubtedly be very interested. Sexual intercourse should be abstained from after vasectomy until test results of a sperm count shows that the semen is free of *all* sperm.

FOLLOW-UP: Test results should be evaluated by a physician if infertility is the problem. The female partner should also be evaluated, since infertility in either partner is often remediable.

CHAPTER 22

Prostate Disease Tests

1. Prostatic Acid Phosphatase (PAP)

2. Prostate Needle Biopsy with
   Malignancy Grading

3. Total Prostate Specific Antigen (PSA)

1. PROSTATIC ACID PHOSPHATASE (PAP)

TYPICAL WORRY: *I have prostate cancer and I worry about whether it has already spread to other parts of my body.*

TEST: Prostatic Acid Phosphatase (PAP)

TEST RESULT: (*example*) 25.0 U/L (SI: same)

URGENCY LEVEL:　　　　　　Action: _√_ Decision: _____

NORMAL RANGE: 0.3-25 U/L (SI: same)

ORIGIN OR SOURCE OF SUBSTANCE TESTED FOR: An enzyme produced by normal and cancerous cells in the prostate gland.

DIFFERENTIAL DIAGNOSIS:

If test results are HIGH:

>　　　　metastasis (spread) of cancer of the prostate gland; benign prostatic hypertrophy (BPH).

If test results are LOW:

>　　　　the spread of prostatic cancer is unlikely (a small or localized metastasis cannot be absolutely ruled out).

COMMENT: Prostatic Acid Phosphatase is not completely specific for cancer of the prostate; a wide variety of diseases, many non-cancerous, may cause elevation of PAP. PAP is *not* useful as a screening test for prostate cancer. It is used primarily to detect evidence of progression of the disease to other parts of the body, especially bone (prostate cancer is a "bone seeker" when it spreads); serial tests may be helpful in monitoring the disease. The test is also used to establish whether or not the tumor has spread beyond the capsule of the gland, and evidence of response of the cancer to therapy.

PAP is tested for in vaginal secretions in cases of alleged rape; the presence of PAP is presumptive evidence that vaginal penetration and ejaculation have occurred (*see Chapter 18, Legal-Issue Tests for more information on this subject*).

FOLLOW-UP: Any elevation of PAP in a patient with prostatic cancer needs to be discussed at length with a physician. Confirmation of spread of the cancer by X-ray, CAT, or other means is important before any decision can be made concerning therapy.

2. PROSTATE NEEDLE BIOPSY WITH MALIGNANCY GRADING

TYPICAL WORRY: *My father and my brother have prostate cancer and so I'm really worried about prostate gland cancer.*

TEST: Needle biopsy of the prostate gland.

(The following is excerpted from Chapter 10, Your Surgical Pathology Biopsy Report)

Prostate cancer is very common in older men. Fortunately, in most men it is slow growing and at times behaves in an indolent manner. Many physicians believe that the Total Prostate Specific Antigen (PSA) test (*see, this Chapter*) is a useful means for detecting prostatic cancer, perhaps early enough to allow prevention of its spread to bones and other organs. It also is useful in monitoring its progression or response to treatment after it has been diagnosed. Detection of cancer using PSA has been very helpful in instituting early treatment. However, great difficulty often arises in the management of a patient with this disease.

Two schemes have been devised to assess the potential behavior of the cancer in relation to the patient's age and in deciding on a choice of therapeutic programs. One of these schemes is *Gleason* scoring. Gleason scoring has been fairly widely accepted as a means of predicting the *prognosis* (how things may turn out) in prostatic cancer. Long-term studies of patients whose prostate cancer has been graded with the Gleason scoring system, i.e., 1 (good prognosis) to 10 (poor prognosis), have shown a strong correlation of the scores with the long-range life expectancy.

Another system of grading of cancer is *conventional* malignancy grading: the tumor's aggressiveness based on the appearance of the cancer cells and their organization as seen through the pathologist's microscope. This grading of prostatic cancer by the two methods allows generalizations about a patient's future outlook when the grades of prostatic cancers (malignancy i-iv, and Gleason 1-10) are combined.

If the pathology report states that cancer of the prostate gland is present and conventional malignancy grade is HIGH (grade iii or iv), and Gleason grade is 8-10:

> poorly behaving malignant tumor: tumor invasion into nearby tissues or distant spread (metastasis) of the cancer is more likely to take place rapidly.

If malignancy grade is INTERMEDIATE (conventional grade ii or iii and Gleason grade 5-7:

> moderately-behaving malignant tumor, but tumor behavior is indeterminate—it may or may not spread rapidly.

If malignancy grade is LOW (conventional grade i, and Gleason grade 1-4):

> well-behaving malignant tumor; the spread of prostatic cancer is less likely to be rapid, if at all.

A problem arises when the scores of either (or both) the Gleason and the conventional scores fall into the INTERMEDIATE category: Gleason 5-7, and conventional ii-iii. Tumor behavior is then less predictable than when scores and grades are either in the HIGH or LOW categories.

Management of prostatic cancer (like breast cancer in a woman) is a difficult and perplexing problem for both the patient, his family, and his doctor because of the complications of various approaches to therapy. The prognosis for a patient with prostatic cancer needs to be discussed at length amongst all three parties involved. The often-heard medical aphorism relating to prostatic cancer is worth remembering: "Prostate cancer is *usually* one that a patient dies with, rather than from." Usually, but surely not always.

(*For more information on Surgical Biopsy Reports, see Chapter 10.*)

3. TOTAL PROSTATE SPECIFIC ANTIGEN (PSA)

TYPICAL WORRY: *My father and my brother have prostate cancer and so I'm really worried about prostate gland cancer.*

TEST: Total Prostate Specific Antigen (TPSA).

TEST RESULT: (*example*) *22.0* ng/mL

URGENCY LEVEL: Action: _√_ Decision: _____

NORMAL RANGE: Thresholds for possible further investigation:

Total PSA:
   Age: 40's: 2.5 ng/mL
           50's: 3.5 ng/mL
           60's: 4.0 ng/mL
           70+: less than (<) 6.5 ng/mL.

ORIGIN OR SOURCE OF SUBSTANCE TESTED FOR: a substance produced only by cells in the prostate gland; total PSA consists of bound-to-protein and unbound-to-protein ("free PSA") fractions.

DIFFERENTIAL DIAGNOSIS:

If test results are HIGH:

   cancer of the prostate gland;
   benign prostatic hypertrophy (BPH);
   inflammation of the prostate gland (prostatitis).

If test results are LOW:

> prostate cancer is unlikely (a small or localized
> cancer cannot be absolutely ruled out);
> post-prostatectomy, or after any other treatment (e.g.,
> radiation) for prostate cancer that has partially
> or completely destroyed the prostate gland;
> falsely low, due to drug therapy for benign (non-
> cancerous) enlargement of the prostate gland
> (BPH); (*see Comment following*).

COMMENT: Some studies have shown that seventy percent of men between the ages of 50 and 70 years have a PSA below 2.0 ng/mL. Low test results may be due to medication (e.g., Proscarä; Avodartä) for prostate enlargement; be sure your doctor is informed if you are taking these drugs.

The rate of change ("velocity") of the PSA over time is significant; an increase of 0.8 ng/mL/year over three years is evidence that cancer may be present even if the test results remain within the normal range. Although PSA testing is useful, there is an appreciable number of false-negative test results (i.e., when the test results fall between the normal range (2.6-4.5 ng/mL) but undetected cancer is present; thus testing annually or every two years is reasonable.

Any rise of the PSA from post-treatment low levels may indicate persistence or recurrence of the cancer.

If the PSA testing is done soon after a digital rectal examination ("DRE") of the prostate gland, there may be further elevation of the test result, but usually only if the test result is markedly elevated to begin with (i.e., >20 ng/mL).

African-Americans and those who have a father or

brother with prostate cancer are considered to be at higher risk for the disease.

Men who have prostate cancer often have reduced free PSA—a fraction of total PSA. If total PSA is only slightly increased, testing for *free PSA* may be necessary. If the ratio of free PSA to total PSA is less than 25%, cancer may be present, and needle biopsy of the prostate gland may be necessary.

FOLLOW-UP: Any elevation of PSA requires consultation with a physician or a surgeon specializing in Urology. Whether immediate treatment or "watchful waiting" is the best course of action is a difficult decision that has to be made by the patient after he has been made aware of the various choices of therapy and the possible complications and consequences of each. The age of the patient at the time the disease is diagnosed, as well as the size of the tumor and whether it is localized or has spread to other parts of the body are important factors that must be discussed at length and in detail with a physician, and with the patient's family before a decision is made concerning which treatment—if any—is best.

CHAPTER 23

Sexually Transmitted Disease (STD) Tests

1. CD4/CD8 Lymphocytes and Ratio

2. HIV-1/HIV-2

3. Rapid Plasma Reagin (RPR)

4. Urethral Culture

5. Vaginal Culture

1. CD4/CD8 LYMPHOCYTE COUNT AND RATIO

TYPICAL WORRY: *I am HIV positive, and wonder if the treatment is helping.*

TEST: CD4/CD8 Lymphocyte Count and Ratio

TEST RESULTS: (*examples*) Total lymphocytes: 1250/cmm.
CD4 lymphocytes: 225/cmm.
CD8 lymphocytes: 296/cmm.
CD4:CD8 ratio: 0.76

NORMAL RANGES: Total Lymphocytes: 1500-4000 /cmm.
(SI: 1.5-4.0x10^9)
CD4: 450-1400/cmm (SI: 4.50-14.0x10^3)
CD 8: 190-725 /cmm (SI: 1.90-7.25x10^3)
CD4: CD8 ratio: 1.0-3.5

URGENCY LEVEL: Action: __√__ Decision: _____

ORIGIN OR SOURCE OF SUBSTANCE TESTED FOR:
Certain types of lymphocytes in the blood, separated by flow cytometry (a special laboratory test). The lymphocyte counts and ratios are indicators of immunodeficiency from *any* cause, including HIV infection.

DIFFERENTIAL DIAGNOSIS:

If Total Lymphocytes are less than 1500/cmm, and/or CD4 Lymphocytes are less than 300/cmm, and/or CD8 Lymphocytes are less than 190/cmm, and the CD4:CD8 ratio is <1.0, HIV is likely, and may be progressing to AIDS.

CHAPTER 23

If Total Lymphocytes are greater than 15000/cmm, and/or CD4 Lymphocytes are greater than 300/cmm, and/or CD8 Lymphocytes are greater than 190/cmm, and the CD4:CD8 ratio is >1.0, HIV is less likely, or if previously diagnosed, is not yet progressing to AIDS.

COMMENT: The Total Lymphocyte count helps your doctor make decisions regarding treatment if you are HIV positive. If you are being treated and test results show abnormalities, your medication may have to be changed. AIDS (acquired immune deficiency syndrome) is a result of HIV infection but may take many months to develop. It has been observed that some individuals apparently develop immunodeficiency disease without known exposure to HIV, but this is quite infrequent.

FOLLOW-UP: Call your doctor if any or all of the above test results are abnormal. Your physician will choose the follow-up tests, if any and any changes in medication that may be necessary.

2. HIV-1/HIV-2 SEROLOGY

TYPICAL WORRY: *I'm afraid I've been exposed to HIV infection.*

TEST: Serologic test for Human Immunodeficiency Viruses (HIV-1 and HIV-2).

TEST RESULT: (*example*) Positive

URGENCY LEVEL: Action: __√__ Decision: _____

NORMAL RANGE: Negative.

ORIGIN OR SOURCE OF SUBSTANCE TESTED FOR: antibodies produced by the body's immune system in response to the HIV infection.

DIFFERENTIAL DIAGNOSIS:

If test results are POSITIVE:

> HIV infection is highly likely, but must be confirmed by a follow-up test (i.e., Western Blot test).

If test results are NEGATIVE:

> infection by HIV is unlikely, but early after exposure the test may be a false-negative.

COMMENT: Most, but not necessarily all diseases associated with this test abnormality are HIV-1 or HIV-2 infections, with or without AIDS (Acquired Immuno-Deficiency Syndrome). The prognosis is better for long time survival if treatment is initiated early. *If the HIV test is negative after the possibility of exposure is presumed, repeating the test in 2 or 3 weeks is essential,* because the antibodies to the HIV virus may not yet have been developed by the body's immune system, but the virus may be present and active in the body.

FOLLOW-UP: If your test results are positive, see your physician immediately. Your physician will choose the follow-up tests, if any, that may be necessary. *Advise your sexual partner(s) of your HIV infection if your HIV test is POSITIVE.*

3. RAPID PLASMA REAGIN (RPR) TEST

TYPICAL WORRY: *I have been sexually active and I suspect my last partner may have a venereal disease.*

TEST: Rapid Plasma Reagin (RPR) Test for Syphilis.

RESULTS: (*example*) Positive.

URGENCY LEVEL: Action: __√__ Decision: _____

NORMAL RANGE: Negative

ORIGIN OR SOURCE OF SUBSTANCE TESTED FOR:
a substance produced by the body in response to syphilis (and other infections).

DIFFERENTIAL DIAGNOSIS:

If the report is POSITIVE:

syphilis; many false-positive reactions, including: autoimmune diseases (e.g., rheumatoid arthritis; systemic lupus erythematosus); pregnancy; old age; viral infection (e.g., infectious mononucleosis, hepatitis); drug addiction; parasitic diseases (e.g., malaria).

If the report is NEGATIVE:

no disease; late stage of syphilis (if clinical history and/or physical findings suggest syphilis).

COMMENT: Syphilis in the acute stage is revealed as a *chancre,* an ulcerative lesion on the genitalia. This acute stage progresses to a secondary stage manifested by a skin rash, followed, often months or years later, by a third stage, often manifested as a non-cancerous brain tumor (gumma), heart valve lesion, or aortic aneurysm. The RPR test varies in the time it becomes positive, and therefore is listed here as an acute disease test. The test has very low specificity, but is more sensitive than a formerly-used screening test, the Venereal Disease Research Laboratory (VDRL) test. Many drugs and a wide variety of infections can cause a *false-positive* RPR test. *A POSITIVE test for syphilis is a panic value in pregnancy.*

FOLLOW UP: A POSITIVE test result requires immediate evaluation by a physician and a follow-up test, usually FTA-ABS. Syphilis is a treatable disease, especially in its early stages. A NEGATIVE test result does not necessarily mean that disease is not present; *false-negatives* can occur, or the disease may be in an early stage, before reagin has been produced by the body. In the late stage of syphilis the RPR is often NEGATIVE.

4. URETHRAL CULTURE

TYPICAL WORRY: *I've had recent unprotected sex with a girl who I thought was clean—but now I have a drip from my penis and it stings when I piss.*

TEST: Urethral bacterial culture (or DNA Detection Test) on the penile discharge fluid.

TEST RESULTS: (*example*) Positive for *Neisseria gonorrheae*

URGENCY LEVEL: Action: _√_ Decision: _____

NORMAL RANGE: Negative, or No growth.

ORIGIN OR SOURCE OF SUBSTANCES TESTED FOR: a bacterium not ordinarily present in the urethra, bladder, or genital organs.

DIFFERENTIAL DIAGNOSIS:

If the bacterial culture is POSITIVE for *Neisseria gonorrheae*:

> definitive evidence of gonorrhea ("the clap"); if the test used was Neisseria gonorrhea DNA Detection Test and the test result was positive, infection is most likely present.

If the bacterial culture is NEGATIVE for *Neisseria gonorrheae*, infection may still be present because of the difficulty in culturing this bacterium, possibly resulting in a false-negative report; if the test used was Neisseria gonorrhea DNA Detection Test and the test result was negative, infection is unlikely.

COMMENT: An urethral culture is taken to detect infection of the male and female sex organs, and it is often referred to as a "Genital Culture". When *Neisseria gonorrheae* infection is present, *Chlamydia trachomatis* may also be present; even if *Neisseria* is not found, *Chlamydia* infection may still be present, often infecting without causing symptoms. If either of these organisms infects a female and is unsuspected, undetected, and untreated, each may cause salpingitis (inflammation of the fallopian tubes), ectopic (tubal) pregnancy, or infertility, or all three.

FOLLOW-UP: Call or see your doctor, who will prescribe treatment and may order additional tests to make sure other sexually transmitted diseases (STD) such as HIV and syphilis are not also present. *Advise any sexual partner of your infection!*

5. VAGINAL CULTURE

TYPICAL WORRY: *I have a heavy and smelly vaginal discharge; I have had herpes infection in the past, and I'm pregnant.*

TEST: Vaginal bacterial/fungal culture of discharge

TEST RESULTS: (*example*) Culture: *Candida albicans*

URGENCY LEVEL: Action: __√__ Decision: _____

NORMAL RANGE: Normal flora; No growth; Negative.

ORIGIN OR SOURCE OF SUBSTANCE TESTED FOR: microorganisms (bacteria, fungi, parasite) not ordinarily present in the vagina and causing infection

DIFFERENTIAL DIAGNOSIS:

If the culture result is POSITIVE:

> for: *Candida,* yeast vaginitis ("thrush", or "the whites"), the most common cause of discharge due to vaginal infection;
> for: *Chlamydia trachomatis; Neisseria gonorrhea; Streptococcus, Group B;* or *Ureaplasma urealyticum:* a bacterial infection by one or more of these bacteria.

If the culture result is NEGATIVE:

> an infecting agent may still be present e.g., viruses such as *Herpes simplex (HSV1 and HSV2)* or *Cytomegalus (CMV)*, or parasites such as *Trichomonas*—which will not be detected by the standard bacterial and fungal

culture techniques but can be detected by "wet mount prep" or Pap smear.

COMMENT: A "wet mount prep" is a quick, inexpensive screening test for *Trichomonas* and *Candida.* Strand Displacement Amplification (SDA) testing and urine cultures may be used in place of the conventional culture of vaginal secretions. Testing for microorganisms can be less expensive when performed or ordered at a Sexually Transmitted Disease clinic.

Teen-agers are often afraid to tell their parents or go to a doctor when they have symptoms or worries about STD. Walk-in Family Planning Clinics (FPC) staffed by friendly and understanding female nurses in a non-intimidating setting are often a solution to this vexing personal, social, (and public health!) problem.

FOLLOW UP: Many infections that are known to be sexually transmitted diseases must be reported to local or state health departments. Treatment for these diseases requires medical expertise, since some untreated STDs may lead to problems of a chronic nature, including infertility.

Call your doctor, who may order other tests to make a specific diagnosis. Newer, highly sensitive tests for many microorganisms are now available that use techniques of molecular biology such as DNA probes. These tests are characteristically more expensive than standard culture tests, but when suspicion of infection is high and usual culture test results are negative, they may be worth the greater expense, given the possible serious complications mentioned above.

CHAPTER 24

Therapeutic Drug Monitoring Tests

1. Activated Partial Thromboplastin
   Time (APTT)

2. Aspirin (Salicylate)

3. Digoxin

4. Lithium

5. Phenytoin (Dilantin)

6. Prothrombin Time (PT) for Anticoagulants

7. Theophylline

1. ACTIVATED PARTIAL THROMBOPLASTIN TIME (APTT)

TYPICAL WORRY: *I'm on heparin as a blood-thinner and now I have had several long nose bleeds. I wonder if my heparin dosage is right.*

TEST: Activated Partial Thromboplastin Time

TEST RESULT: (*example*) 50 seconds (SI: 50 seconds)

URGENCY LEVEL: Action: __√__ Decision: _____

NORMAL RANGE: 25-39 seconds (SI: 25-39 seconds)

ORIGIN OR SOURCE OF SUBSTANCE TESTED FOR: the patient's blood plasma, tested to discover specific blood clotting factor deficiencies as well as the effectiveness of an anticoagulant (blood thinner).

DIFFERENTIAL DIAGNOSIS:

If test results are HIGH:

> the dosage of the anticoagulant (heparin) may be too high, and bleeding may occur somewhere in the body.

If test results are LOW:

> the dosage of anticoagulant (heparin) is unlikely to lead to abnormal bleeding, but may be too low to be effective in preventing blood clots from forming.

COMMENT: If the test result is HIGH, the dosage may be at a level where acute internal or external bleeding is likely. If the test result is LOW, the dosage may be insufficient to prevent thrombosis (blood clotting in a blood vessel)—which is most likely the reason heparin was prescribed. The test is also used to identify deficiency of certain factors in the blood (there are many such factors) that might be causing abnormal bleeding problems such as black-and-blue areas in the skin.

FOLLOW-UP: If your test results are either HIGH *or* LOW (above or below the Normal Range), notify your doctor at once.

2. ASPIRIN (SALICYLATE)

TYPICAL WORRY: *I'm taking a large amount of aspirin for my arthritis and I wonder if it's causing the dizziness and ringing in my ears I have.*

TEST: Serum salicylate

TEST RESULT: (*example*) 80mg/dL (SI: 3.6mmol/L)

URGENCY LEVEL: Action: _√_ Decision: _____

THERAPEUTIC RANGE

> For blood clotting prevention (e.g., stroke and heart attack): 10 mg/dL (SI: 0.72 mmol/L)
> for pain relief: 15-20 mg/dL (SI: 1.09-1.45 mmol/L).

ORIGIN OR SOURCE OF SUBSTANCE TESTED FOR: any over-the-counter (OTC) medication containing aspirin (e.g. coated or uncoated aspirin, Anacin™, Ascriptin™, Bufferin™, Ecotrin™, Empirin™).

DIFFERENTIAL DIAGNOSIS:

If serum salicylate is HIGH:

> Overdose of aspirin

If serum salicylate level is LOW:

> Dosage may be too low to either relieve pain or reduce inflammation.

COMMENT: Signs of aspirin toxicity (poisoning) include dizziness, tinnitus (ringing in the ears) and other symptoms and signs of a nervous system disorder. Enteric (coated) low-dose aspirin (81 mg, "children's aspirin", "St. Joseph's Asprin™") is often prescribed by doctors as one measure to help prevent heart attacks; its effect is to prevent or discourage blood platelets from clumping together to cause a blood clot inside a blood vessel such as a coronary artery. Low-dose aspirin is unlikely (when taken once a day) to cause toxicity or stomach problems such as ulcers or bleeding. In young children both acute and chronic aspirin overdose is dangerous and can be fatal.

FOLLOW-UP: See your doctor if results are HIGH or LOW. He or she may order that the test be repeated, and/ or your medication dosage and schedule be adjusted. There are many causes of dizziness, not the least of which is an impending stroke. If your dizziness or ringing in your ears persist, consult your doctor!

3. DIGOXIN

TYPICAL WORRY: *I worry about everything. Now I'm worried that my heart medicine dosage isn't right, because my heart beat seems to be irregular.*

TEST: Digoxin

TEST RESULT: (*example*) 2.9 ng/mL (SI: 3.7 nmol/L)

URGENCY LEVEL: Action: __√__ Decision: _____

THERAPEUTIC (EFFECTIVE) RANGE: 0.8-2.0 ng/mL (SI: 1.10-2.6 nmol/L)

ORIGIN OR SOURCE OF SUBSTANCE TESTED FOR: a drug that is used in the treatment of heart disease (e.g., heart failure or irregular rhythm).

DIFFERENTIAL DIAGNOSIS:

If blood Digoxin is HIGH:

> possible overdose of Digoxin (i.e., more than is necessary or desirable to control symptoms).

If blood Digoxin is LOW:

> not enough blood level of Digoxin to be effective in treating some forms of heart disease.

COMMENT: Digoxin at a level higher or lower than your doctor has intended for your treatment should be corrected immediately. Improper levels occur in the blood for many reasons. Commonly occurring reasons include taking the wrong number of pills, taking them on an incorrect schedule, forgetting to take the pills, failure of your body to metabolize (utilize, or break down) the drug normally, or on occasion due to an incorrect prescription. Laboratory testing for Digoxin blood levels is important for the control of symptoms of heart failure or irregular heart beat.

FOLLOW-UP: Call your doctor immediately if your Digoxin is out of therapeutic range; your doctor will want to check your medication prescription and your adherence to the schedule for taking the pills, and to check your heart and your body for signs of trouble.

CHAPTER 24

4. LITHIUM

TYPICAL WORRY: *I have developed blurry vision and I have twitching of my muscles. Could it be related to the lithium drug I'm taking?*

TEST: Lithium

TEST RESULT: (*example*) 2.3 mEq/L (SI: 2.3 mmol/L)

URGENCY LEVEL: Action: __√__ Decision: _____

THERAPEUTIC RANGE: 0.6-1.2 mEq/L (SI: 0.6-1.2 mmol/L)

ORIGIN OR SOURCE OF SUBSTANCE TESTED FOR: a medication used in the treatment of bipolar (manic-depressive) psychiatric disorder.

DIFFERENTIAL DIAGNOSIS:

If the Lithium level is HIGH:

> overdosage of the medication.

if the Lithium level is LOW:

> probable insufficient dosage, below effective therapeutic level.

COMMENT: Any underdosage symptoms (returning manic-depressive behavior) or symptoms of overdosage (see below) should be reported to a physician, since symptoms of overdosage may occur at any dosage level, *including therapeutic levels.*

Table 9

Symptoms of overdosage at various levels

Serum level mEq/L (SI: mmol/L)	Symptoms
1.5-2.5	dizziness, blurred vision, weakness, frequent urination
2.6-3.0	restlessness, muscle twitching, loss of urine control, coma
> 3.0	seizures, death.

FOLLOW-UP: Contact your doctor if test results are either HIGH or LOW. He or she may order that your medication dosage and/or your schedule for taking the drug be adjusted.

5. PHENYTOIN (DILANTIN™)

TYPICAL WORRY: *I've been taking Dilantinä medication for seizure control ever since I was a child and I know that I need to have the dosage checked because I've noticed double-vision again.*

TEST: Serum Phenytoin (Dilantinä)

TEST RESULT: (*example*) 25 mg/mL (SI: 99 mmol/L)

URGENCY LEVEL: Action: __√__ Decision: _____

THERAPEUTIC RANGE: 10-20 mg/dL (SI: 40-79 mmol/L).

ORIGIN OR SOURCE OF SUBSTANCE TESTED FOR: a medication used in the treatment of seizure disorders (e.g., "epileptic fits").

DIFFERENTIAL DIAGNOSIS:

If the serum phenytoin level is HIGH:

overdose of the medication.

If the serum phenytoin level is LOW:

dosage may be too low to be effective, and seizures may occur.

COMMENT: Symptoms of over-dosage of phenytoin at various levels include unsteadiness, double vision, involuntary side-to-side eye movement, and dizziness. Allergic reactions to the drug may also occur, Any symptoms of over-dosage should be reported to a physician, since symptoms of over-dosage may occur at any dosage level, *including therapeutic levels.* Under-dosage may lead to recurrence of seizures. Small changes in dosage can have marked clinical effects. Theophylline and some antidepressant medications may affect the test result, so your physician should be reminded if you are taking these other medications.

FOLLOW-UP: Periodic check-ups with a physician are important for anyone on anti-seizure medication. Part of the check-up should be monitoring of the serum levels of phenytoin.

CHAPTER 24

6. PROTHROMBIN TIME (PT) FOR ANTICOAGULANTS

TYPICAL WORRY: *I have been taking my blood-thinner for a long time because of my thrombophlebitis. I haven't had my pro-time checked in quite a while.*

TEST: Prothrombin time (PT)

TEST RESULTS: (*example*)

> Patient: 58 seconds
> Control: 11.5 seconds

URGENCY LEVEL: Action: __√__ Decision: _____

SIGNIFICANT VALUES:

> Control range: 10-13 seconds
> Therapeutic range: 2 to 3 times Control
> Panic range: > 3 times Control

ORIGIN OR SOURCE OF SUBSTANCE TESTED FOR: clotting factors in the blood, produced in the liver.

DIFFERENTIAL DIAGNOSIS:

If the results are ABOVE the therapeutic range (effective treatment level):

> possible overdose of the anticoagulant (blood-thinner).

if the results are BELOW the therapeutic range:

possible insufficient anticoagulant in the blood to prevent abnormal blood clotting; drug interaction (e.g., antibiotics and warfarin)

COMMENT: This is a simple and inexpensive test, widely used for many years as a means of monitoring the adequacy or inadequacy of levels of anticoagulants in the blood such as heparin, but especially when coumarin and warfarin are used over a long term. The test is run and reported in comparison to a normal control (blood from a patient or a substance not altered by the use of an anticoagulant).

FOLLOW-UP: See your doctor if test results are either HIGH or LOW. He or she may order that the test be repeated or your medication dosage and/or your schedule for taking the drugs adjusted.

7. THEOPHYLLINE

TYPICAL WORRY: *I have been taking theophylline medication for my asthma and I want to check my dosage because I'm wheezing.*

TEST: Serum Theophylline

TEST RESULTS: 26 µg/mL (SI: 146 mmol/L)

URGENCY LEVEL: Action: __√__ Decision: _____

THERAPEUTIC RANGE: 10-20 ug/mL (SI: 56-111 mmol/L)

ORIGIN OR SOURCE OF SUBSTANCE TESTED FOR: A medication used in the treatment of asthma and chronic obstructive pulmonary disease (COPD).

DIFFERENTIAL DIAGNOSIS:

If the Theophylline level is HIGH:

> prescription overdose of the medication;
> reactive overdose due to:
> > heart failure; a severe infection; liver disease;
> > use of birth control pills.

If the Theophylline level is LOW:

> dosage may be too low to be effective (i.e., wheezing may recur).

COMMENT: Any symptoms of under-dosage or over-dosage should be reported to a physician, *immediately if there is over-dosage.* Nausea and vomiting, anorexia, heart arrhythmias, abdominal pain are but a few of the many signs and symptoms of toxicity which can lead to death. Theophylline can decrease the levels of phenytoin and lithium in the blood.

FOLLOW-UP: Theophylline levels should be monitored periodically by a physician because of the severity of reactions that can occur from overdose. Remind your physician if you haven't been scheduled for a review of your medication.

AFTERWORD

"Every man is the builder of a temple, called his body, to the god he worships after a style purely his own, nor can he get off by hammering marble instead. We are all sculptors and painters, and our material is our own flesh and blood and bones."

Henry David Thoreau

T horeau, the rustic American philosopher had it right more than one hundred fifty years ago. Socrates also had it right more than twenty four hundred years ago when he said that the unexamined life is not worth living. His words, like Thoreau's, still ring true, and we can rightly paraphrase those words today:

"The unexamined *body* is not worth living *with*".

In the Army I was told that if you were to teach anything to a GI, you should tell him what you are about to say, say it, and then tell him what you said. Although my Army career is long in the past, this Afterword follows the same spirit. The Table of Contents told you what I was going to say, Parts I, II and III said it, and the Afterword is a précis of what I said to refresh your memory and to emphasize the book's message.

Recall the before-the-mirror self-appraisal described in Chapter 1. That daily quick examination of the *outside* of your body, its weight, appearance and profile is worhtwhile, but consider the aphorism of an English biologist of the last century, T.H. Huxley: "The great end of life is not knowledge but action". Don't just stand there, do something! What you should do is examine the *inside* of your body. That's what laboratory tests do. But it's *your* responsibility to use them and the counsel of your healthcare provider.

And it's important to remember that although all the laboratory tests in the armamentarium of medicine will not keep you always well or disease-free, a healthy life-style and continual self-examination will go a long way towards a protracted and productive life, assuming that like most of us, you have been dealt a good genetic hand by your parents.

Taking responsibility for your own health is an often overlooked imperative of wellness. Choosing a good diet, vigorous exercise, adequate sleep; resistance to the temptations of addicting drugs, smoking, and drinking alcohol in excess; simple safety measures like using seat belts, using headgear whenever your body is susceptible to head injury, and avoiding recreation where the dangers of serious permanent injury outweight peer pressure and the temporary endorphin "high" of the sport—all of these will help keep you well, and save you money throughout life.

A useful way to keep in touch with changes and advancements in medical, health, nutrition, and wellness knowledge is to subscribe to one or more newsletters devoted to these subjects. Authoritative and reliable information can be found in many of these scientifically oriented newsletters that are written in a style that is both interesting and understandable. Several of the distinguished medical institutions in the United States such as Johns Hopkins Medical Institutions, Harvard Medical School, University of California Medical School at Berkeley, the Mayo Clinic, the Cleveland Clinic, Tufts University School of Nutrition, and others offer their newsletters at affordable prices. You may have already been solicited! Johns Hopkins' *Health After 50* has also published a consumers guide to a variety of tests, and The University of California at Berkeley has an encyclopedia of wellness. Each of these publications can be usefull additions to a home health library.

For those who are computer literate, an excellent website relating to clinical laboratory tests and health care can be found at: *http://labtestsonline.org/understanding/analytes/cbc/test.html.*

Much of what you have found in this book, and more, is on this easy-to-navigate site.

Share responsibility for your health with a competent healthcare provider, one who will order the proper immunization and necessary laboratory tests as part of an annual health examination to assure that things are going well inside your body. Then when the unavoidable and unanticipated overtake you, or if you happen to be by nature one of the worried well, perhaps referring to the contents of this book will help you understand those laboratory tests you or your doctor has ordered or the surgical pathology reports you have received. And I hope the messages here have been useful in getting you to a laboratory for either physician-ordered or direct access testing on your own.

Here is something else to keep in mind. Laboratory science is always evolving. Newer, better tests continually show up. Furthermore, not all professionals agree on every subject, which is very important for the advancement of science. A basic tenet of scientific inquiry is to continually suspect, doubt, challenge, and debate what is printed in scientific journals and books—including this one.

Remember again Dr. Kassirer's words . . . "*Medical imperialism is obsolete.*" And remember, too, that you are paying for your test results, either directly or indirectly, and you should not be intimidated into accepting limited information—or none—about your health. It's your body and it's your blood, with all the rigths, responsibilities, and privileges of ownership. And *you* are in charge of the warranty!

And here is a last warning: if *you* ever receive an *Action* test result in a laboratory report, do not postpone doing something right away. Call your physician or healthcare provider at once!

INDEX

A

action level 40
activated partial thromboplastin
    time (APTT) 175, 341, 342
acute appendicitis 47, 48
acute gastroenteritis 47
acquired immunodeficiency
    syndrome (AIDS) 283, 332
adenocarcinoma 61, 100, 102,
    161, 204
adenomatous polyp 102
adenoma 100
adrenal gland 30, 296
alanine aminotransferase (ALT)
    111, 127, 243
alcohol 71, 289, 290
alkaline phosphatase (ALP)
    111, 127, 243, 245
alpha1-fetoprotein 303, 304
American Cancer Society 52
American Heart Association 44, 52
anemia 30, 184-188
anemia profile 30
annual physical checkup 34
antigen 198, 314
antigenic protein 198
antiglobulin 314
apolipoprotein A and B 70,
    261, 264-266

arthritis profile 30
aspartate aminotransferase
    (AST) 111, 127, 243
aspirin 341, 345

B

basal cell 100
benign prostatic hypertrophy
    (BPH) 61
benign tumor 100
bladder infection 45, 47
blood-loss anemia 185
blood sugar. 148, 226, 251-2,
    281-2
blood urea nitrogen (BUN) 234
blood vessels 100
body burns 189
bone marrow 100, 102, 185,
    189
bone-marrow disease 185
breast 102
bulimia 188

C

C-reactive protein 115, 219, 261,
    264, 268
Campylobacter pylori 228
Canadian Task Force 52
Candida albicans 141, 144

carcinoembryonic antigen (CEA) 197, 198. *See also* tumor marker
carcinoma 100
carcinoma-in-situ (CIS) 100, 102, 104, 204
cardiac risk 151, 261, 267, 269
CAT scan 50
CD4:CD8 lymphocyte count and ratio 330, 332
cervical cancer 104
cervix 102
chemotherapy 61, 185, 201, 259
Chlamydia trachomatis 143, 146, 338, 339
chloride 303 *See* sweat test
cholesterol 148, 149, 152
chorionic gonadotropin 303, 311
chronic-disease anemia 173, 186
cobalamin 177
colon 102
colon cancer 52, 104, 160
colposcopy 162, 205
complete blood count (CBC) 178, 180, 181
conjugated bilirubin 111
conjunctivitis 24
creatine kinase (CK) 262, 275. *See also* creatine kinase MB fraction (CK-MB)
creatine kinase MB fraction (CK-MB) 261, 272
creatinine 234
creatinine clearance 235
cryotherapy 106
cystic fibrosis 222, 224, 306
cystic fibrosis DNA content 223, 225, 307
cystitis 45, 144, 145

D

deciliter (dL.) 37, 68
decision level 39
dehydration 154, 179, 189
Department of Health and Human Services 44
depression 80
diabetes 172, 230, 248
diarrhea 117, 133
differential diagnosis 44, 51
digoxin 271, 341, 347
Dilantin. *See* phenytoin
direct bilirubin 125
direct-access testing (DAT) 23, 26, 73
diuretics 189
diurnal rhythm 43
diverticulosis 47
DNA probe 147, 340
drug monitoring 341, 355
ductal adenoma 102
ductal carcinoma 100, 102

E

ectopic pregnancy 47, 48, 310
electrophoresis 184, 190
enzyme systems 43
erythrocyte sedimentation rate (ESR) 116, 219
erythropoietin 185
estrogen receptor assay (ERA) 103, 197, 200. *See also* progesterone receptor assay
estrogens 299, 301

F

false positive 42, 216
fasting blood sugar (FBS) 70, 168, 252, 282

fertility. *See* infertility
forensic 292, 294

G

gallbladder 125
gallbladder attack 47
gamma glutamyl transferase
  (GGT) 112, 127, 243
gastritis 228
genital culture 146, 339
Giardia lamblia 118
Gleason scoring 104, 105, 324
glucose 37, 281
gonorrhea 219, 337
gout 27, 259
grade i, ii, iii, iv 100

H

heart attack 189
Helicobacter pylori 228
hematocrit 153, 178
Hemoccult 148, 203
hemoglobin 178, 184
hemoglobin C. *See* hemoglobin
  C disease
hemoglobin C disease 189, 190
hemoglobinopathies 184, 189
hemolysis 189
hemolytic anemia 186
hepatitis panel 111, 119
herpes virus 80
heterophil 50, 111, 120
high-density lipoprotein
  (HDL). *See* high-density
lipoprotein cholesterol
  (HDLC) 149, 150, 261
high-density lipoprotein
  cholesterol (HDLC) 149,
  150, 261
homocysteine 261, 264, 268

hormone replacement therapy
  (HRT) 162, 205
human immunodeficiency
  disease (HIV)
  111, 122, 212, 232, 330
Huxley, Thomas H. 44, 358
hypertension 31, 247
hyperthermia 189
hypoglycemia 38, 227

I

infection 336, 337, 340
infectious mononucleosis
  50, 111, 120, 124
infertility 143, 147, 283, 303,
  318, 320, 338, 340
invasion 100

J

jaundice 111, 119, 126

K

Kassirer, Jerome 25, 28, 62, 359
keratosis 103
kidney cancer 52

L

lactic dehydrogenase (LDH)
  112, 127, 243
lead poisoning 157
leukemia 100, 179, 185
  lymphocytic 101
  monocytic 101
  myelogenous 101
libido 297
lipoma 102
liters 68
lithium 341, 348
liver disease 125, 126
local extension 101

low-density lipoprotein (LDL). *See* low-density lipoprotein cholesterol (LDLC)

low-density lipoprotein cholesterol (LDLC) 150, 261

lower limit 37

luteinizing hormone 299, 301

Lyme disease serology 112, 131

lymph nodes 101, 102

lymphatics 101

lymphocytes 155, 180

M

macrocytic anemia. *See* megaloblastic anemia

magnetic resonance imaging (MRI) 50, 106

malignant tumor 101, 259

mammogram 35

McBurneys point 47

mean corpuscular hemoglobin (MCH) 153, 178, 184

mean corpuscular volume (MCV) 153, 178, 184

medical imperialism 25

megaloblastic anemia 182, 187

melanoma
  malignant 106

mesenteric lymphadenopathy 47, 48

metastasis 101, 105

metastatic 101, 102

mg/dL 68, 69, 289

microalbuminuria 213, 248

microcytic 187

micromols 68

milligram (mg.) 68

milliliters (ml.) 68

millimols (mmol.) 68

mono. *See* infectious mononucleosis

Monospot 121, 124

multiple sclerosis (MS) 50

N

Neisseria gonorrheae 338, 339

nonalcoholic fatty liver disease (NAFLD) 245

normal ranges 36, 38, 69

normal results 26, 38, 39

nurse practitioner 297

nutritional anemia 173, 188

O

occult blood 70, 104, 148, 160, 197, 203

osteoarthritis 218

osteocalcin 213, 250

osteoporosis. *See* osteocalcin

ovarian cyst 47, 48

over-the-counter tests (OTC) 26

overweight 168, 252, 282

P

panels 54

Pap smear 104, 147, 162, 197, 206, 340

Papanicalou. *See* Papanicalou smear maturation index

Papanicalou smear maturation index 299, 300, 302

papilloma virus 80

parasites 137, 146, 339

parentage 291, 292

paternity 282, 291, 292

pathologist 97

pathology 97

pelvic inflammatory disease (PID) 47, 48

penile discharge 337
per deciliter 67
per liter 67
pernicious anemia. 187 *See*
    megaloblastic anemia
phenytoin 341, 351
picomols 68
platelet count (plt) 178, 179, 189
polycythemia vera 189
polyp 101, 102
porphyria 47
postprandial 168, 252, 282
pregnancy 182, 254, 284, 303,
    311, 313
progesterone receptor assay
    (PRA) 103, 197, 201
prostate 102, 164, 207, 235, 293,
    321, 322
prostate cancer 104, 106, 323,
    324, 326
prostate-specific antigen (PSA)
    104, 148, 166, 197, 210,
    321, 324, 327, 329
prothrombin time (PT) 111,
    126, 127
protocols 201
psoriasis 218
psoriatic arthritis 218
pyelitis 45
pyelonephritis 45

R

random blood sugar 148, 168,
    213, 252, 282
rape 292, 293
rapid plasma reagin (RPR)
    112, 135, 213, 254, 330, 336
red big toe 259
red-blood-cell count 153, 178
reference ranges. *See* normal
    ranges

reticulocytes 190
rheumatoid arthritis (RA) 115,
    120, 134, 255, 335
rheumatoid factor (RF) 213,
    255
ruled out 45, 49

S

salicylate 341, 345. *See* aspirin
sarcoma 101
screening tests 34
semen analysis 71, 303, 320
senile keratosis 103
sensitivity 51. *See also* specificity
sentinel node 101
serum iron 173, 195
sexually transmitted disease
    (STD) 80, 276, 284, 330
shift to the left 49
sickle cell. *See* sickle-cell
    anemia
sickle-cell anemia 173
sickle-cell crisis 189
skin 103
smear review 155, 180
solar keratosis 103
specificity 51
sputum 211
sputum cytology 71
squamous cell 101
squamous-cell carcinoma
    102, 106, 204
stool for ova 112, 132
sugar 168
surgical excision 106
surgical pathology report 97
sweat test 212, 222, 303, 307
symbols
    mg/L 67, 68, 198, 304
    mmol/L 67, 68, 346, 350
syndrome 60

Systeme Internationale (*SI*) 67
systemic lupus erythematosus
    (SLE) 134, 214, 215, 218,
    242, 253, 256, 335
systems review 23

T

T-4 257
target cells 190
test groups 54, 55
testosterone 295, 296, 298
thalessemia 189, 190
theophylline 260, 341, 354,
    355
thrombocythemia 154, 179
thrombocytopenia 155, 180
thyroid stimulating hormone
    (TSH) 80, 148, 169, 170
thyroid storm 257
thyrotoxicosis 257
tired all the time;tired override
    50, 169
tissue specimen 97
total bilirubin 111, 127, 243
total cholesterol (TC) 276, 287
triglycerides 261, 265
troponin 261, 273, 275
tumor 102
tumor marker 198

U

UA with micro. *See* urinalysis
    with microscopic exam
ulcerative colitis 137
upper limit 37, 257
urethral caruncle 45
urethral culture 112, 143, 330,
    338
urethritis 45
uric acid 27, 213, 218, 260

urinalysis with microscopic
    exam 148, 172, 234
urinary tract 144, 145, 235
urine culture 45, 112, 145, 147,
    238, 340

V

vaginal culture 112, 330, 339
vasectomy check 320
venereal disease (VD) 283
virus 113, 139, 141

W

watchful waiting 40, 166, 209,
    329
website 359
within normal limits 36
worried well 14, 24

X

X-ray 249

Y

yellow jaundice 119